Rakhimova Feroza
Sabirova Sabohat
Sanzharbek Rakhimberganov

Information technologies in medicine

Rakhimova Feroza
Sabirova Sabohat
Sanzharbek Rakhimberganov

Information technologies in medicine

Study guide

ScienciaScripts

Imprint

Cover image: www.ingimage.com

This book is a translation from the original published under ISBN 978-3-659-60271-9.

Publisher:
Sciencia Scripts
is a trademark of
Dodo Books Indian Ocean Ltd. and OmniScriptum S.R.L publishing group

120 High Road, East Finchley, London, N2 9ED, United Kingdom
Str. Armeneasca 28/1, office 1, Chisinau MD-2012, Republic of Moldova, Europe
Printed at: see last page
ISBN: 978-620-8-31810-9

Contents

Research Editors:
Rakhimov Bakhtiyar Saidovich- Head of the Department of Biophysics, Physical Culture and Sports of Urgench Branch of Tashkent Medical Academy, Candidate of Technical Sciences
Sabohat Kabulovna Sabirova Sabohat Kabulovna- Assistant of the Department of Biophysics, Physical Education and Sport, Urgench Branch of Tashkent Medical Academy
Rakhimova Feroza Bakhtiyarovna- Assistant of the Department of Biophysics, Physical Education and Sport, Urgench Branch of Tashkent Medical Academy
Rakhimberganov Sanzharbek Rustamovich - 6th year medical student of Urgench branch of Tashkent Medical Academy.
Reviewers:
Madatov H.A.- Head of the Department of Information Technologies of Urgench State University, Ph.
Yusupov P.N.- Urgench branch of TATU named after P.N. Muhammad al-Khwarizmi, Associate Professor of Engineering Sciences Department, Ph.

Methodical instructions to practical works on the subject "Information technologies in medicine" for full-time students of specialities 60910200 - "Medical Business", 60910300 - "Paediatric Business", 60910400 - "Medical and Preventive Business".

The process of formatting documents, methods of creating text styles, automatic table of contents, work with graphics, as well as tables and diagrams in Word are considered in detail. In the MS Excel section the question of creating spreadsheets, working with formulas, functions, diagrams, making reports is considered. Problems on search of solution, selection of parameter are analysed.

Descriptions of practical exercises with general theoretical information, test questions and assignments, in accordance with the programme and the list of recommended literature.

The collection will assist teachers in organising practical work, and may also be useful for students when repeating the material studied and preparing for credit.

Introduction

The collection of practical works is compiled in accordance with the working programme for the discipline "Information technologies in medicine" for the specialty: 60910200 - "Medical Business", 60910300 - Pediatric Business", 60910400 - "Medical and Preventive Business"

Practical works occupy a central place in the study of computer science discipline. Their purpose is to organise and manage the student's independent work in the course of laboratory and practical classes, as well as:

- formation of practical skills in MS Word, MS Excel, MS Access, Paint, MS Power Point;
- generalisation, deepening, systematisation and consolidation of the theoretical knowledge gained;
- formation of skills to apply the acquired knowledge in practice;
- development of such professionally significant personal qualities as observation, ability to compare, generalise, independence, responsibility, creative initiative.

As a result of laboratory and practical works the student should: ***know:***

- basic concepts of automated information processing;
- basic system software products and application software packages;

be able to:

- use the learnt application software tools.

The collection of practical classes consists of an explanatory note, a description of practical works, which are provided with general theoretical information, control questions and tasks in accordance with the programme and a list of recommended literature.

Before starting work the student must familiarise himself with the theoretical material and know the *safety regulations*:

1. Be attentive and careful. Follow the teacher's instructions precisely.
2. Do not switch on the computer without the teacher's permission;
3. Carefully study the progress of the work before it is done;
4. Switch on the PC in sequence: uninterruptible power supply unit, monitor, system unit;
5. Do not keep foreign objects, including mobile phones, in the workplace;
6. Do not touch the display screen, do not touch the wires;

7. When working on a PC, the screen should be 55-60 cm from the eyes, perpendicular to the gaze;
8. Do not move around the room while working on the PC. Avoid sudden movements;
9. Switch off the PC when the work is finished.

A certain number of hours are allocated for each practical work.

The form of student reporting is specified for each practical work.

It is recommended to work on a computer running Windows XP operating system, in the text editor MS Word, in the tabular processor MS Excel, in the DBMS MS Access, in the graphic editor Paint, in the programme for creating multimedia presentations MS Power Point.

The collection will help teachers in the organisation and management of independent work of students in the process of laboratory and practical classes, and students can use the manual when repeating the studied material, preparing for the exam.

When carrying out practical work, attention should be paid to: the **requirements for carrying out practical work:**

1. Study the theoretical material.
2. Answer the theoretical questions.
3. Organise the tasks in a workbook for practical work.

Reporting Form:

When carrying out practical work, it is necessary to:

- write down the number and topic of the class;
- write down the assignment;
- describe the performance of the work;
- answers to self-check questions.

Practical work No. 1

ORGANISATION OF WORK ON A PC. Work with the PC keyboard

Purpose of the lesson. To learn how to initially organise work on a PC, switch on/off the PC, learn how to work with the PC keyboard.

Type of work: frontal

Lead time: 2 hours

Equipment: PC, notebook

The chronological map of the lesson is 80 minutes.

Organisational part: cleanliness of premises, equipment, sanitary and hygienic conditions.

Student attendance is 2 minutes.

Assessment of students' knowledge : brief overview of the subject, questions and answers with students - 10 minutes.

Setting a new theme - 20 minutes.

Determination and consolidation of the level of mastery of the subject - 35 minutes.

Test questions - 10 minutes.

Homework - 3 minutes.

Practical work requirements:

1. answer the theoretical questions
2. organise the tasks in the practical workbook

Theoretical material

When you switch on your computer, the lights should light up, the monitor should make the same sound as when you switch on the TV, and the power supply fan in the system unit should make a noise.

The operating system starts automatically after the PC is switched on with the Power button on the system unit. The PC first checks that its main devices are working properly, then you may have to enter the user password or network password if the PC is connected to a network.

After booting the Windows environment, the so-called Desktop appears on the screen, with *the Taskbar* at the bottom of the Desktop in a standard installation. On the left side of the taskbar is the *Start* button.

The Main Menu structure includes two sections: mandatory and arbitrary. The user can set the items of the arbitrary section at will. Sometimes such items are created automatically when installing applications (e.g. Ms Office).

The main part of the screen is occupied by *the Workspace.* It contains icons - *My Computer, My Documents, Internet Explorer, Recycle Bin,* corresponding to the folders of the same name. Folder shortcuts can also be located there. The set of icons and shortcuts is chosen by the user, so their number and list may vary.

The fixed capitalisation mode is activated by pressing the [Caps Lock] key and the [Caps Lock] indicator will light up. Attention! Do not confuse with the [Num Lock] key, which enables the numeric keypad.

Task 1.1. Switching on the PC. Starting work on the PC

Work order

1. Switch the PC on, press the power button on the monitor, press the power button on the system tray

Press the Power button on the unit.

2. Wait for the operating system to boot (approximately 60 s).

3. Study the composition of the Windows *Main Menu.* Click the *Start* button to open the Windows *Main Menu.* Explore the commands in the mandatory Windows *Main Menu* section - *Run, Help, Find, Setup, Documents, Favourites, Programs.* Note that shutting down your computer is done with the *Shutdown* command.

4. Examine the appearance of the screen and the basic icons *of the Workspace.*

Task 1.2. Entering information using the keyboard

Work order

1. Take a close look at the keyboard of a personal computer.

2. To display the information entered from the keyboard, open the electronic notepad. To do this: click the *Start* button, select *Programs*, then *Standard,* then *Notepad.*

3. Turn on the numeric keypad with the [Num Lock] key (the [Num Lock] indicator will light up) and type the digits from 1 to 9, after typing the digits, press the Enter key. Note that the cursor has moved down one line.

4. Locate the tab key [Tab] on the keyboard. Type a sequence of numbers separated by an interval by pressing the [Tab] key: 123 456 789. After typing the numbers, press the enter key [Enter].

5. Set the Russian keyboard layout. To do this, on the screen on the right side of the taskbar, find the EN/RU indicator and set the RU position corresponding to the Russian language.

6. Examine the basic text keyboard. Find the keys for the letters fywa and OLJ.

7. Assume the starting position of your hands on the keyboard with the four fingers of your left hand (except for the thumb) resting on the fywa keys and the four fingers of your right hand (except for the thumb) resting on the ALJ keys. Round your fingers as if you were holding a large apple in each hand.

Place your thumbs over the intermediate key, which is the largest key below the letter keys. The intermediate key makes spaces between words. If a word ends with a letter on the left, the right thumb strikes the intermediate key, and vice versa.

The keys should be pressed one by one, the impact should be even and equal in strength on each key.

8. Check that the [Caps Lock] indicator is not lit. If necessary, switch it off with the [Caps Lock] key.

9. Type fywa and OLDJ, separating the words with a space.

10. At the end of each line of input characters, press the Enter key.

11. Press the [Caps Lock] key that locks capital letters. The [Caps Lock] indicator should light up. Type fywa and OLDJ. Note that the text is typed in capital letters. Memorise the purpose of the [Caps Lock] key. Switch off the [Caps Lock] indicator.

12. Press in turn all the keys (from left to right) in the top row with numbers from 0 to 9 and other characters. Press [Enter] to move to a new line.

13. Locate the [Shift] key on the keyboard that changes the dialling case. Press Shift and, without releasing it, press all the top row keys in turn again. Note that different characters from the previous set are printed.

14. Set the Latin keyboard layout. To do this, find the EN/RU indicator on the right side of the taskbar and set the EN position.

15. Press the [Shift] key and, without releasing it, press all the top row keys in turn again.

Note that some characters are again different from the previous set(Fig.1.1).

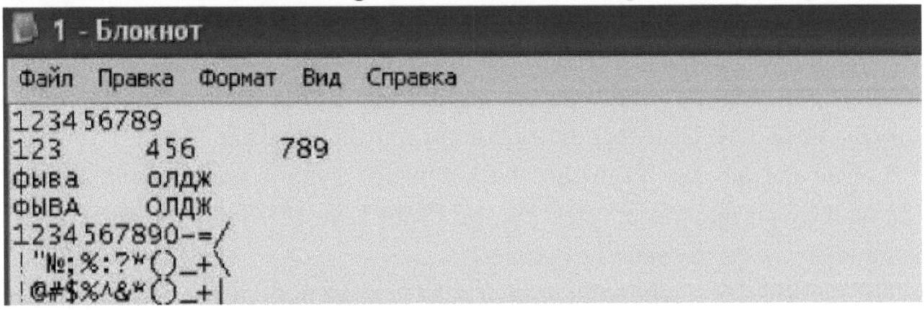

1 - Блокнот

Файл Правка Формат Вид Справка

```
123456789
123        456        789
фыва       олдж
ФЫВА       ОЛДЖ
1234567890-=/
!"№;%:?*()_+\
!@#$%^&*()_+|
```

Fig 1.1 Character set in the electronic notepad

16. Place the cursor on the first line at the very beginning of the character set and press the A key several times (seven to eight times). You will see *fff* characters appear, as we have the Latin keyboard layout set and the Caps Lock indicator off.

17. Delete the digits to the right of the typed letters *fffff* by pressing the Delete key on the keyboard. Note that the digits to the right of the cursor are deleted.

18. Press the Back Space key (left arrow above the Enter key) that deletes characters to the left of the cursor. Delete all *fffff* characters to the left of the cursor.

19. Go to the very end of the typed characters by pressing the Ctrl and End keys simultaneously (press the Ctrl key and, without releasing it, press the End key). Go back to the beginning of the text by pressing the Ctrl and Note keys simultaneously. Memorise these keyboard shortcuts.

20. Locate the cursor keys (in the form of arrows) on the keyboard and move the cursor left/right across the row and up/down across the rows.

21. Find the *Close* button (with a cross) in the upper right corner of the *Notepad* window and click on it. The programme will display a warning window with the text "The text in the Untitled file has been changed. Do you want to save the changes?". Click the Yes button.

22. Open your existing keyboard simulator and use it to practise your PC keyboard typing skills.

23. Switch off the computer. Click the *Start* button in the taskbar with the left mouse button, select Shutdown from the main menu. In the dialogue box that appears, tick the command.

24. Switch off the computer and click *OK.*

25.

Additional tasks

Practising the skills of entering information using the keyboard.

To perform the exercises, open *Notepad.* Learn the rules of typing before starting the exercises.

Typing rules. When typing on the keyboard, the hands move first of all, and with them the fingers, which should always be next to each other. When typing, the fingers do not move apart at all: the hands move up, down and sideways, and the fingers move together, with the right finger striking the right key.

The starting position for hands on the PC keyboard is shown in Fig. 1.2: four fingers of the left hand (except the thumb) are placed on the fywa keys; four fingers of the right hand (except the thumb) are placed on the OLDJ keys; thumbs are placed over the intermediate key (space bar);

all fingers except the thumbs should be slightly rounded (as if you were holding a large apple in each hand);

Always return your fingers (hands) to the starting position after striking the keys.

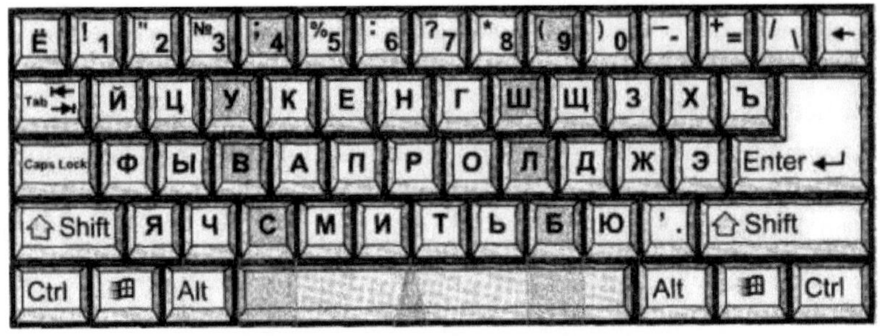

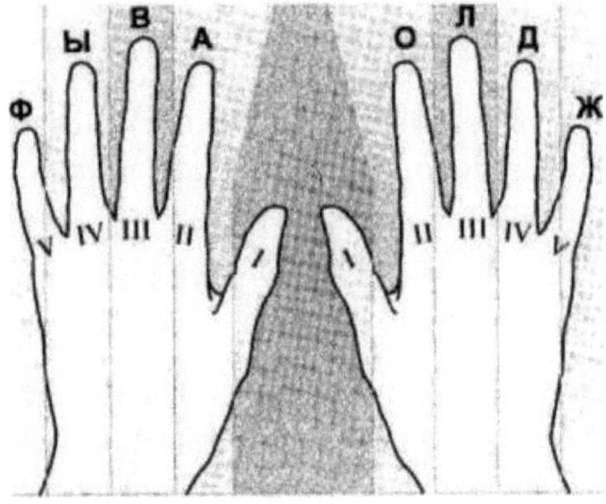

Fig. 1.2 Starting position for hands on the PC keyboard

Task 1.3. Keep the hands in the starting position of the middle row stationary and type the text of the exercise

aaaaaaaaaaaaaaaaaaaaaaaaaaaaaaввввввввввввввввввввввввввввв ы ы ы ы ы ы ы

y y y y y y y y y y y y y y y y y y y y y y y y y y y y y y y y y y y y y y y y y y y y y y y y y y y y y y y y y y y y y y y y y y y y y y y y y y y y y y y y y y y y y y y y y y y y y y y y y

ave ave ave ave ave ave ave ave ave ave ave ave ave ave ave ave ave ave ave ave ave ave ave ave ave ave ave ave ave ave ave ave ave ave ave ave ave ave ave ave ave ave ave ave ave ave ave ave ave ave ave ave ave ave ave ave ave ave ave ave ave ave ave ave ave ave ave ave ave ave ave ave ave ave ave ave ave ave ave ave ave ave ave ave ave ave ave ave ave ave ave ave ave ave

ould ould ould ould ould ould ould ould ould ould ould ould ould ould ould ould ould ould ould ould ould ould ould ould ould ould ould ould ould ould ould ould ould ould ould ould ould ould ould ould ould jodlo fywa jodlo fywa jodlo fywa avyf fywa avyf fywa avyf fywa avyf fywa avyf fywa avyf fywa avyf fywa avyf fywa avyf fywa avyf fywa avyf fywa avyf fywa

Task 1.4. Type the text of the exercise, returning the hands to the starting position

wa ool

аааооо ааоао оааоо аоаоа ооаоа ао оао аоаао аоаоа ао аоа вввооо ввово воовв оввоо вова вова вовво ововo вова вова лллввв ллвлв вллвв лвлвл ввлвл вал влвлв вол лов олово ааалллл аалал лаалл алала lalla alla alla alla allo lava lvlv vova oolol lololol lolo lolo vol

fy j

ыыыддд ыыдыд дыыдд ыдыды ддыды ад два вода воды ыддыы дыдыд ода вола вдова выводы доводы лады дылда фффддд ффдфд дффдд фдфдф ддфдф фа даф фдффд фдфдф фал фол лафа фалды жжжддд zhjddfdf zhjf zhjf zhjf zhjf zhjf zhjf zhjf zhjf zhjf zhjf zhjf zhjf zhjf zhjf zhjf zhjf zhjf zhjf zhjf zhjf zhjf zhjf zhjf zhjf zhjf zhjf zhjf zhjf zhjf zhjf zhjf zhjf zhjf zhjf zhjf zhjf zhjf zhjf zhjfфыф ыыфыф дыф фалды дджджж жддж жажджа дввважды джджд жжджд ждал додж фдфыж дды ыффж фжыыд ад ода два дылыда выжал доводы фол вожжа жало ждал додж жажда фа лыжа выжал выводы фалды ложа вдова ждала лафы дважды

mi ti

мммттт ммтмт тммтт мтмтм ттмтм вот вам мыло мттммт тмтмт латы фото флот фата лом том атом там мат мото жмот иииттт иитит тиитт итити ттити идти тиф итиит титит вита фитиль лифт ломти таити ььиии ььиьи иььии иьиьи ииьиь лить вить ьиььи иьиьи доить жить мылить жалить mmmmуу уу ууууууу тьтьт ььтьт вымыть толь выжить молоть итимь тмььи титм мтиiь мьмит ьитмь вылить молоть молитва выжить дымить фитиль фильм тьма ломать.

Reporting Form:

When carrying out practical work, it is necessary to:

- Write down the number and topic of the class.
- Write down the assignment.
- Describe the performance of the work in detail.
- Answer the control questions.

Supervisory Questions:

1. Describe the procedure for switching on the computer.
2. How does the operating system boot up?
3. What appears on the monitor screen after the operating system boots?
4. How do I view the Main Menu?
5. What is included in the mandatory section of the main menu?
6. What do you know about the arbitrary section of the main menu?
7. What is a working field?
8. What icons are located on the workspace?
9. How do I start the Notepad programme?
10. How do I switch on the numeric keypad?
11. What happens on the keyboard after the numeric keypad is turned on?
12. Which key should I press to move the cursor to a new page in Notepad?
13. How do I switch the keyboard layout to English?
14. Which key must be pressed to enable fixed capitalisation mode?
15. What happens when you press the key combination CTRL+END, CTRL+HOME?
16. Describe the procedure for shutting down the computer.

Recommended reading: 1.1,1.2, 2.2.

Practical work No. 2

ORGANISING WORK IN THE WINDOWS ENVIRONMENT. CREATING AND DELETING SHORTCUTS

Objective of the lesson. Studying the technology of organising work in the Windows environment.

Creating shortcuts, working with the Recycle *Bin.*

Type of work: frontal

Lead time: 2 hours

Equipment: PC, Microsoft Office

The chronological map of the lesson is 80 minutes.

Organisational part: cleanliness of premises, equipment, sanitary and hygienic conditions

hygienic conditions.

Student attendance is 2 minutes.

Assessment of student knowledge: brief overview of the course, questions and answers with students - 10 minutes.

Setting a new theme - 20 minutes.

Determination and consolidation of the level of mastery of the subject - 35 minutes.

Test questions - 10 minutes.

Homework - 3 minutes.

Practical work requirements:

1. answer the theoretical questions
2. organise the tasks in the practical workbook

Theoretical material

The window in which the user is currently working is called the *active window.* The active window is placed in the foreground on top of the other windows. Any command refers to the active window, which operates in priority mode.

By grabbing and moving the window border with the mouse, you can resize the window. By grabbing the window title with the mouse, you can move the window. Toolbar is an optional element of the window, it contains icons and buttons intended for quick access to the most frequently used commands. You can add a toolbar from the *View* menu using the *Toolbar* command.

Scroll bars on the right and bottom of the window allow you to move vertically and horizontally when the window borders do not allow you to see the entire contents of the window.

When working with several windows, the easiest way to switch to another window is to click on the visible part of the window. If the windows are expanded to the whole screen, you can switch to another window by one of the following methods: by clicking on the button with the window name in the taskbar or by pressing the [Alt] and [Tab] keys (a window with icons of running programmes will open in the middle of the screen; without releasing the [Alt] key, press the [Tab] key).

To change the window width, move the mouse pointer to the vertical side of the window. The pointer will look like a horizontal double-headed arrow. Drag the window edge horizontally to the side and the window will shrink.

To change the window height, move the mouse pointer to the top or bottom sides of the window, and the cursor will look like a vertical double-headed arrow. Drag the edge of the window and the window dimensions will change in height.

To change the window height and width simultaneously, move the cursor to the corner of the window - the mouse pointer will turn into a diagonal double-headed arrow. By dragging the window frame diagonally, you will reduce the window size.

To organise, right-click on the free part of the taskbar (where the Start button is located) and select the *Cascade* windows command from the context menu so that only the window titles are visible. To view the contents of all open windows at the same time, select the Windows from *top to bottom* or *Windows from left to right* command.

To create a shortcut, place the cursor on an empty space on the desktop and right-click (right-click). In the context menu that appears, select the *Create/Label* command. In a standard installation, the full file path to the MS Word launcher file is: C:/Program Files/ Microsoft Office/ Office 11/ WinWord.exe.

The Recycle *Bin* is located on the desktop and is used to temporarily store deleted files. It allows you to recover files deleted by mistake. Files deleted from floppy discs are not placed in the Recycle *Bin*. Clearing the Recycle *Bin* deletes files and frees up memory in your computer. Before defragmenting the disc, only special programs can recover files.

To recover deleted files from the Recycle Bin, select the name of the object to be recovered and choose the *Recover* command from the *File* menu. If you need to recover several objects, select their names while holding down the [Ctrl] key.

All objects are deleted from the Recycle *Bin using the File/Empty Recycle Bin* command.

Explorer is a software tool that provides access to local and network resources. The purpose of Explorer is to display the contents of folders; open, copy, move, delete, rename folders and files; launch programmes; display the contents of the folder tree on the screen. To open it, right-click on the Start / Explorer button or select Start / Programs / Standard / Explorer.

Task 2.1. Repeat the exercise that you did in practical session 1. To do this, run the Baby Type shortcut (20 min.) Task 2.2. Operations with windows in the Windows environment Work order 1. Switch on your computer. Wait until the Windows operating system has finished loading. *2.* From the desktop, double-click the *My Computer* shortcut to open two windows in sequence: *My Computer* and *C: Drive.*

Notice that two buttons corresponding to these windows appear in the taskbar. 3. Examine the main elements of the window. Locate the following window elements on the screen: - borders - frames that limit the window on four sides, title bar located under the upper border of the window. - window control buttons - *Collapse, Restore, Close* (on the right side of the title bar); - menu bar located below the title bar. The menu provides access to the basic set of commands; - the toolbar (buttons of basic operations). 4. Make the *My Computer* window active and explore the process of minimising/unmodifying windows. Expand the window to the full screen using the *Expand* button - *the* window will increase in size and occupy the entire desktop. The *Expand* button will turn into a *Restore* button with two overlapping squares. Clicking on the *Restore* button returns the window to its previous appearance. 5. By moving the windows (behind the window header) and changing the linear dimensions of the windows (vertical and horizontal), arrange the windows sequentially in five variants according to the sample (Fig. 2.1).

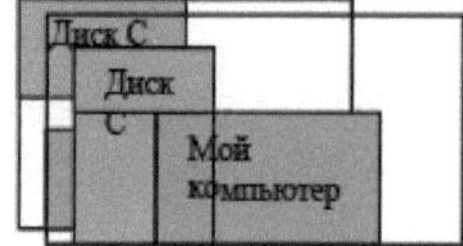

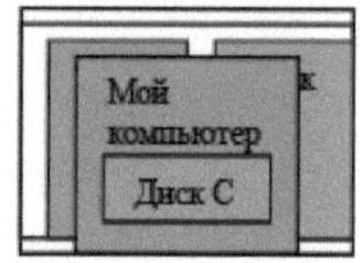

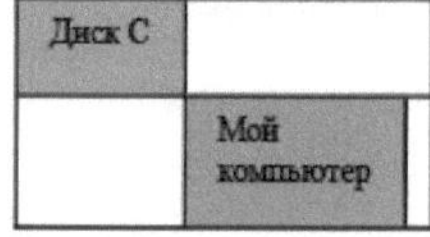

Fig. 2.1. Variants of windows arrangement on the monitor screen

6. Organise the windows on the screen.

7. Close the *My Computer* and *C: Drive* windows (*File* menu, *Close* command by pressing [Alt]+[F4] keys simultaneously or by clicking the Close window button*).*

Task 2.3. Creating shortcuts

Work order

1. Create a shortcut for the Microsoft Word text editor on the desktop. (Figure 2.2).

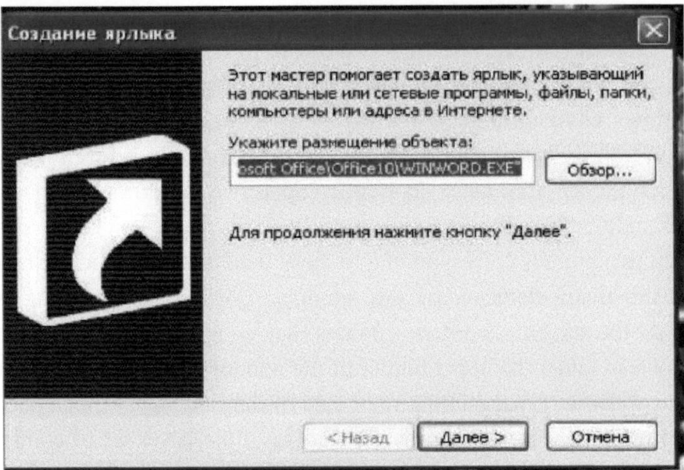

Fig. 2.2. Creating a shortcut

2. In the command line of the *Create Shortcut* window, enter the file path to the launching file of the Microsoft Word programme - WinWord.exe. You can use the *Browse* button. Click the *Next* button to continue.

3. The next window prompts you to select the name of the programme as the shortcut name or replace it with another name. Leave the suggested name. Click the *Done* button. MS Word shortcut appears on the desktop.

4. Change the appearance of the created shortcut. By right-clicking on the shortcut (cryptogram) of the Word programme, call the *Shortcut Properties* window (Fig. 2.3).

Change the cryptogram, to do this go to the *Label* tab, click on the *Change icon* button. Select your favourite type of shortcut icon and confirm your choice.

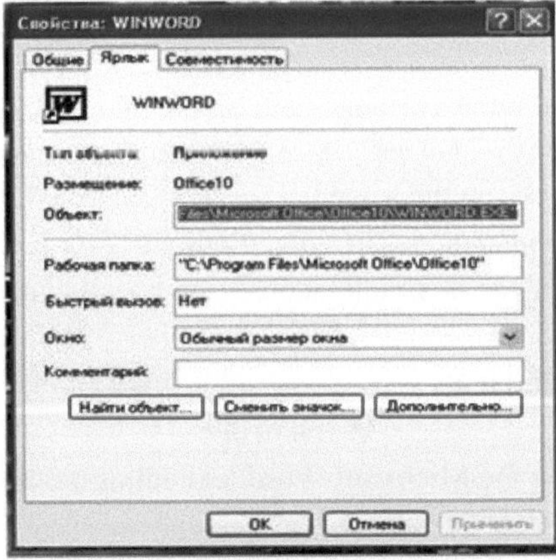

Fig. 2.3 Shortcut property window

Change the cryptogram, to do this go to the *Label* tab, click on the *Change icon* button. Select your favourite type of shortcut icon and confirm your choice.
5. Delete the shortcut you created to the Recycle *Bin* by dragging the shortcut to the Recycle *Bin* icon with the mouse.

Task 2.4. Technology of work with the "Basket" window

Work order

1. Open the Recycle *Bin* window and view its contents.

To do this, double-click the Recycle *Bin* icon on the desktop. In the *View* menu, set the *Table* command (Fig. 2.4). Examine the properties of the deleted shortcut - type, size, deletion date.

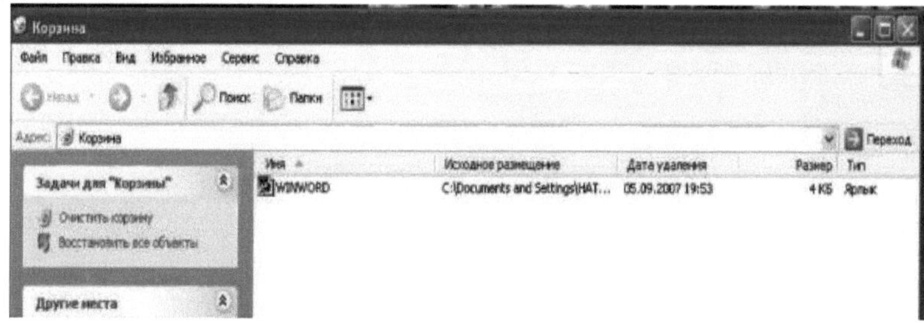

Fig 2.4. Basket window

2. Restore the deleted shortcut to the desktop.
3. Perform a complete cleaning of the Recycle *Bin.* Call the properties of the Recycle *Bin* by right-clicking on its icon and select (left-click) the *Clear Recycle Bin* command in the context menu that opens.
4. Change the size of the Recycle *Bin.* After right-clicking the *Recycle Bin* icon, select the *Properties* command. In the window that opens, set the slider to corresponding division - 10% of the disc capacity (Fig. 2.5).

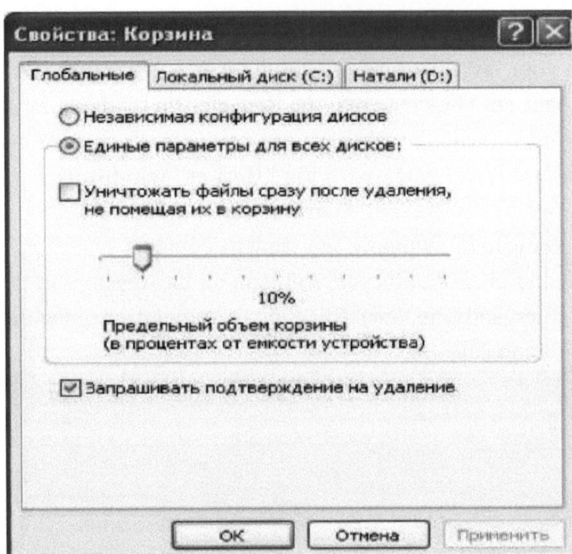

Figure 2.5. Change of the basket capacity

Additional task

Task 2.5. Create a shortcut on the desktop for the MS office programme Excel (C:/Program Files/Microsoft office/Office 11/excel.exe)

Check to see if the programme you have selected has a different cryptogram icon.

Change the view of the shortcut. Delete the shortcut to the *Trash. Restore the shortcut.*

Task 2.6. Start the Notepad text editor from the Explorer programme.

Task 2.7. Create a document "Freshers' debut" with the following text:

Dear freshers!

You are invited to attend the Freshman Debut celebration!
Which will be held on 27 September 2011 at 15.00 in the auditorium of IPTI.

We look forward to seeing you!

Task 2.8. Save the document with the name "Freshers' Debut" in the folder My Documents/ ETET-11-9-1/ Ivanov**

Task 2.9.

1. **Copy a text file from Explorer to the desktop**
2. **Launch the Explorer programme and open the My Documents folder**
3. **Rename the Freshman Debut file to the Invitation file using the context menu.**

Reporting Form:

When carrying out practical work, it is necessary to:

- Write down the number and topic of the class.
- Write down the assignment.
- Describe the performance of the work in detail.
- Answer the control questions.

Supervisory Questions:

1. Which window is called the active window?
2. How is the active window positioned on the workspace?
3. How can I change the size of the window?
4. How do you move a window?
5. How do I add a Window Toolbar?
6. How do you go from one window to another?
7. What do I need to do to organise the windows?
8. Describe the procedure for creating a shortcut.
9. What is a basket?
10. What happens after I delete files from the Recycle Bin?
11. Files deleted from floppy disks are placed in the recycle bin?
12. What ways do you know of to recover deleted files from the Recycle Bin?
13. How can I clear my shopping basket?
14. What is a conductor?

Recommended reading: 1.1,1.2, 2.2.

Practical work No. 3

CUSTOMISING THE WINDOWS USER INTERFACE. MY COMPUTER" WINDOW

.

BASICS OF GRAPHIC IMAGE PROCESSING

Purpose of the lesson. Formation of skills of setting up the operating system, user interface, working parameters, study of methods of creation and processing of graphic images by means of standard programmes.

Type of work: frontal

Lead time: 2 hours

Equipment: PC, Paint

The chronological map of the lesson is 80 minutes.

Organisational part: cleanliness of premises, equipment, sanitary and hygienic conditions.

Student attendance is 2 minutes.

Assessment of student knowledge: brief overview of the course, questions and answers with students - 10 minutes.

Setting a new theme - 20 minutes.

Determination and consolidation of the level of mastery of the subject - 35 minutes.

Test questions - 10 minutes.

Homework - 3 minutes.

Practical work requirements:

1. answer the theoretical questions
2. organise the tasks in the practical workbook

Theoretical material

The Control Panel allows you to customise the look and feel of your computer, install and uninstall programs, set up network connections and user accounts.

Double-clicking the *Date/Time* icon on the control panel opens a window for setting the date and time parameters. The same can be achieved by double-clicking the time indicator icon on the taskbar. The date and time set on the computer's system clock are recorded when you finish working with a document and help you find the latest version of the file.

The screen properties window contains several tabs: *Background,* Screen saver, *Appearance, Settings.* Background allows you to decorate the part of the desktop that is free of windows and icons with a background pattern or pictures (wallpaper) from the available wallpaper.

The Place switch in the Centre position places the drawing in the centre of the screen. *The Place* switch in *the Centre* position places the drawing in the centre of the screen, in the *Multiply* position it repeats the drawing repeatedly across the entire workspace. The screen saver (screen saver) is selected from the screen saver list. The computer idle time, after which the screen saver appears, is set in minutes in the *Interval* list.

My Computer provides a universal program that provides quick access to local computer resources, network drive, various devices (printer, discs) and their configuration. Activating the *My Computer* icon opens a window with icons corresponding to the local or network resources of your computer. To copy a file, select it and choose *Copy* from the *Edit* menu. To paste a copied file, place the cursor at the paste location (highlight your folder) and select *Paste* from the *Edit* menu. To delete a folder, you can use right-click on the system menu button of the bus folder.

Assignment 3.1. Using the Windows Control Panel to configure settings

Work order

1. Open the Control Panel (Fig.3.1). Ways to open the *Control Panel:*

- open the My Computer folder and click on *Control Panel;*
- click the *Start* button and select *Setup/Control Panel* from the main menu.

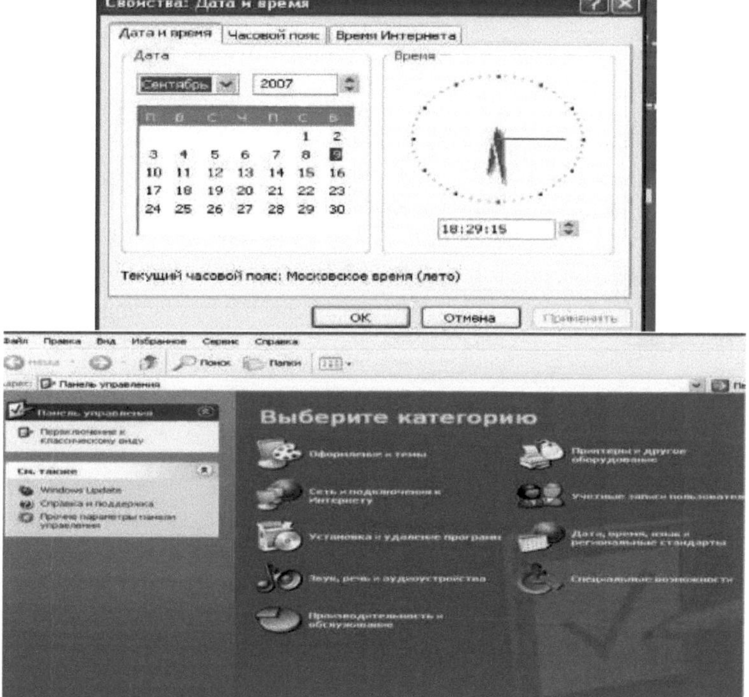

Fig.3.1 Control panel

2. Set the current date and time of the computer's system clock at the time of the exercise, as well as our time zone (Fig. 3.2).

Fig.3.2 Setting the date, time and time zone

3. In the "Keyboard" folder window (click the Control Panel *Keyboard* icon) on the *Speed* tab set the speed of repetition and flicker of the cursor, as well as the interval before the start of repetition and character (Fig. 3.3).

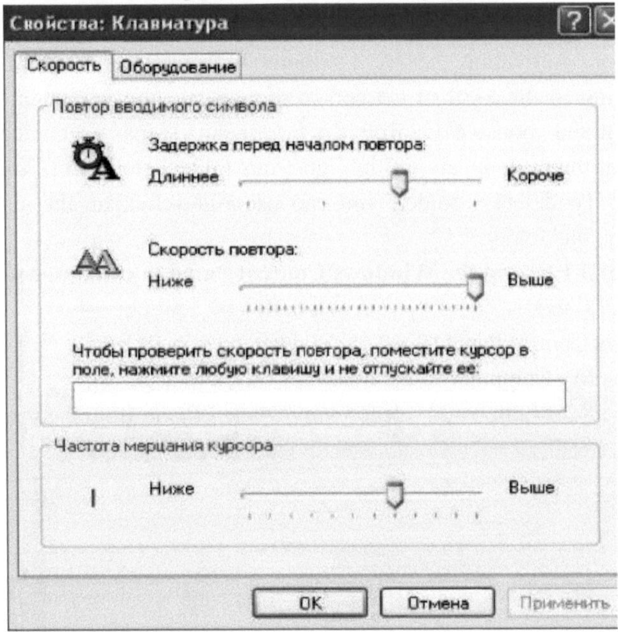

Fig.3.3 Setting the repeat and flicker speed of the cursor

4. In the *Mouse* window (*Mouse Buttons* tab*)* set the configuration "for right-handed" (or "for left-handed" if you are left-handed) and set the optimal speed of double-clicking the mouse buttons (you can check it by clicking in the test area) (Fig. 3.4).

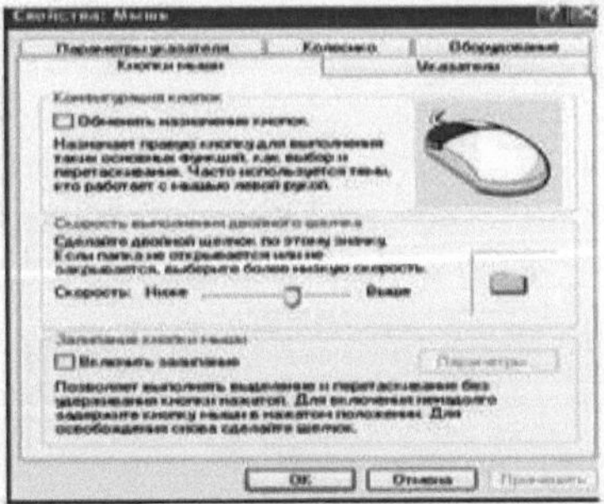

Fig. 3.4. Setting the properties of the computer mouse

On the Pointer Options tab, select *Move and* define a trail behind the mouse pointer. Note how the trail follows the mouse pointer.

Note: Mouse and keyboard settings on some computers, depending on the design type, may be located in the *Control Panel* in the *Printers and Other Hardware* folder. 5. Configure the screen. Open the *Properties: Screen* dialogue box by double-clicking the *Screen* icon in the Control Panel or by right-clicking the mouse after placing the pointer on a free desktop surface. 6. Set the background you like. 7. Set the screensaver you like and set the interval to 5 min. 8. On the *Design* tab select your favourite design from the list of standard schemes created by designers (Fig. 3.5).

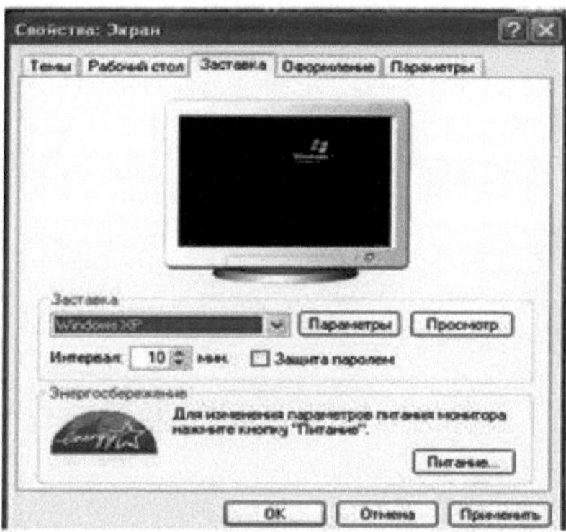

Fig. 3.5. Selecting the screen design

Task 3.2. Setting the folder content viewing style

Work order

1. Open the *My Computer* window. Set the view style *to Large Icons (View/Icons)*. Use the *View* menu to set the view styles *Icons, List, Table, one by one.* Note the difference between the view styles of the folder contents.
2. Sort the contents of the My Computer folder. For sorting in the tabular viewing style, click on the headings: *Name, Type, Full size, Free.* Note that clicking on a heading again will sort the parameter in reverse order.
3. To sort in other styles (non-table styles), execute the *Organise Icons* command from the *View* menu and set the sort key (by name, file type, size or date).

Task 3.3. Copying, moving and deleting files (folders) in the My Computer window

Work order

1. Create a new folder on the C: drive. To do this, select the C: folder icon in the *My Computer* window and activate it by double-clicking it. Select

File/Create/Folder, name the folder (use your last name as the folder name) and press [Enter].

Note. If you want to create a new folder inside another folder, first select the folder with the mouse and then create the new folder.

2. On the C: drive, find the smallest file by size. To do this, in the C: drive window, set the tabular viewing style *(View/Table)* and sort the files by size.

3. Copy the largest file you found to your folder using the *Edit/Copy* and *Edit/Paste* commands.

4. Search the C: disc for all files with the ehe extension. To search, open the search window *(Search),* set the search mask *.ehe and search area - disc C: (Fig. 3.6), then click the *Find* button.

Note. If you enter a keyword in the document name, all documents with this word in the name will be found.

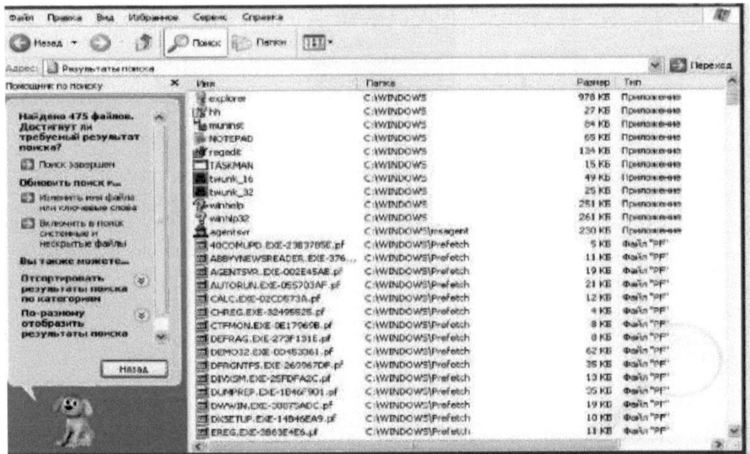

Fig.3.6. Search for files with *.ehe extension on the C drive:

5. Search the C: drive for all files with the .doc extension. To search, open the search window *(File/Find),* specify the search mask *.doc and the search area - disc C:.

6. Copy four of the found files to your folder.

7. Create a shortcut to your folder on the C: drive. To do this, place the cursor on the folder and use the *File/Create Shortcut* command.

8. Copy your folder shortcut to the desktop by dragging and dropping it from the C: drive window while holding down the [Ctrl] key.

9. After the teacher has checked your work, delete your folder and its shortcut. To delete a folder, file or shortcut, select the icon with the mouse and use the *File/Delete* command.

Task 3.4. Open the Trash folder, find the deleted shortcut and folder and

restore them

Task 3.5. On the *Move* tab of the *Mouse* window, remove the loop behind the mouse pointer

Task 3.6. Restore the default screen settings

Assignment 3.7. Study the interface of the Paint application

Work order

1. Launch the built-in graphic editor - the standard Paint programme *(1StartProgramsStandardPaint).* Expand the application window to the full screen.

2. Study the appearance of the Paint window. Start by reviewing elements common to all Windows programmes: title bar, system menu buttons, window control buttons - *Collapse, Restore, Close.*

3. Examine the *Toolbar* buttons. If the toolbar is not on the screen, open it with the *View/Toolbar* command. Select each tool with the mouse and move the mouse pointer to the workspace. Notice how the appearance of the mouse pointer changes.

Explore the *Colour Palette.* If the colour palette is not on the screen, call it with the *View/Palette* command (Fig. 3.7). Find the area where the current colour is displayed. Note that the current colour (upper square) is selected in the Colour Palette with the left mouse button, and the background colour (lower square) is selected with the right mouse button.

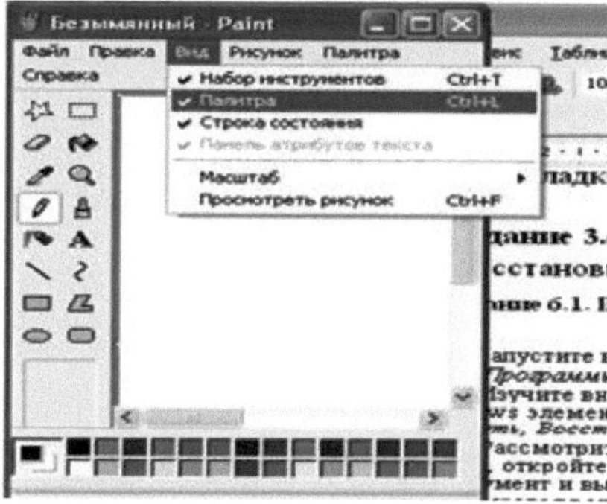

Fig. 3.7. Paint application window

Assignment 3.8. Studying the techniques of creating drawings in Paint

Procedure 1. Having chosen the shape of a geometric figure (rectangle), draw several rectangles with multi-coloured background fills (Fig. 3.8).

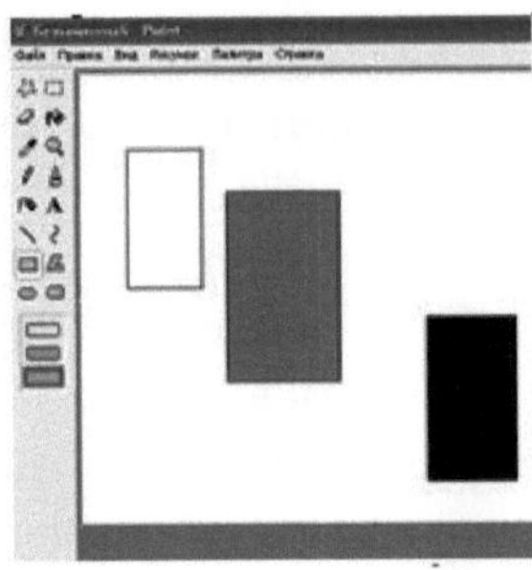

Fig.3.8. Creation of geometrical figures with filling

Below the set of tools there are options for selecting the type of shape, the upper one specifies a contour rectangle of contour colour, the middle one - a coloured rectangle (contour colour - current, fill colour - background), the lower one - the "inside" of the rectangle without a contour line (background colour). Select the shape border colour by clicking the left mouse button in the palette (black), the background colour by clicking the right mouse button (white, blue, black).

Save the drawing in your folder with the name "Sample Drawing 1". 2. Using the toolbar options, draw a cup of coffee with milk (Figure 3.9). To colour the drink in the cup, create a new colour - "coffee with milk".

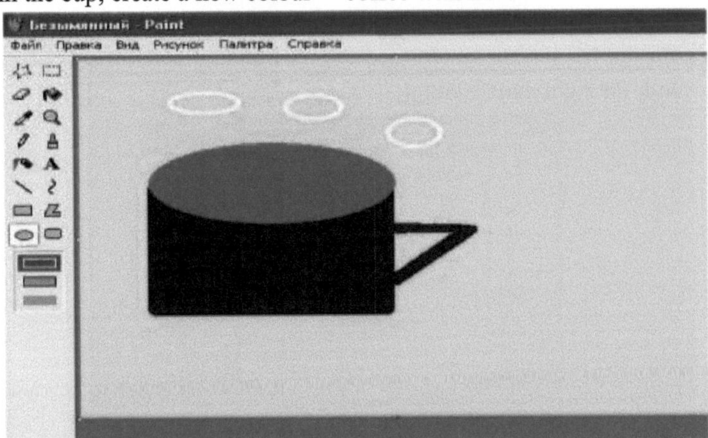

Figure 3. 9. Creating a drawing using Paint

3. To create a new colour (coffee with milk) in the palette, select the *Palette/Modify Palette* command *(Figure 3.10)*. In the upper part of the dialogue box there is the *Base colour palette.* To define a new colour, select the closest colour from the base palette and click the *Define Colour* button; the rainbow colour definition matrix will open on the right side of the window (Fig. 3.11). Select any node on the right side of the colour matrix with the mouse, and then adjust the brightness using the bar on the right side of the matrix (move the

mouse). When you are satisfied with the new colour, click the *Add to Set* button, and the new colour will be added to the additional colour palette.

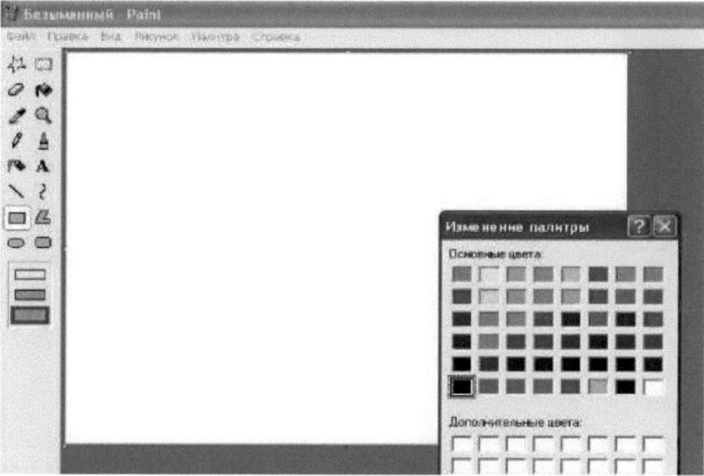

Fig. 3.10. Base and additional colours of the palette

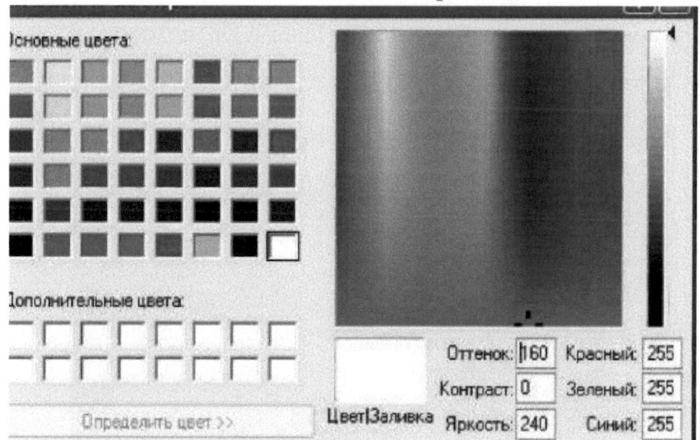

Fig. 3.11. Creating a new additional colour

Save the created drawing in your folder with the name "Sample Drawing 2".

4. Setting a multi-coloured background, draw three regular coloured circles. Remember that pressing the Shift key allows you to draw the correct geometric shapes.

5. Copy the three circles. To copy, select the drawing fragment *with the Selection* tool. Click the *Selection* button of the toolkit and stretch a dotted rectangle around the selected fragment with the mouse. After selection use the *Edit/Copy* and *Edit/Paste* commands (Figure 3.12).

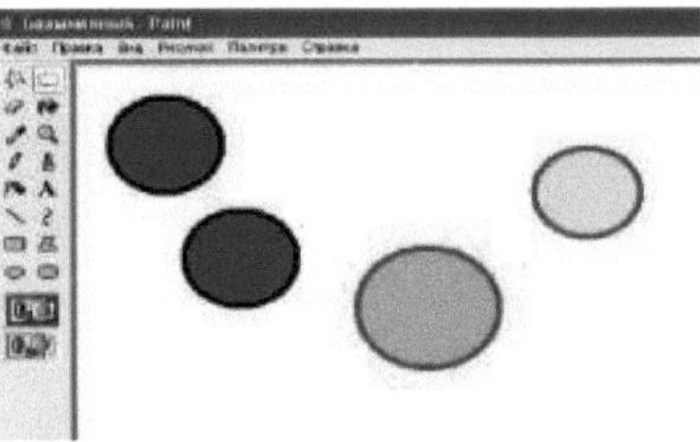

Fig. 3.12. Demonstration of fragments copying and rotation options

6. Rotate the fragment of the drawing. Select the fragment *with the Selection* button, rotate it with *the Reflect/Rotate* command of the *Drawing* menu.

7. Enter the text "Copy and rotate drawings" using the *Inscription* tool.

8. Save the drawing in your folder with the name "Sample Drawing 3".

Assignment 3.9. Inserting drawings into Paint from a file

Work order

1. Paste your existing picture from a file (you can paste a picture from the Windows folder) using the *Edit/Paste from* file command (specify the file type - point drawing *.bmp) (Fig. 3.13).

2. Enter the text there. To do this, click the letter A on the toolbar.

You can change the font type, size, etc. To do this, activate the Text Attributes Panel (*View/Text Attributes Panel*).

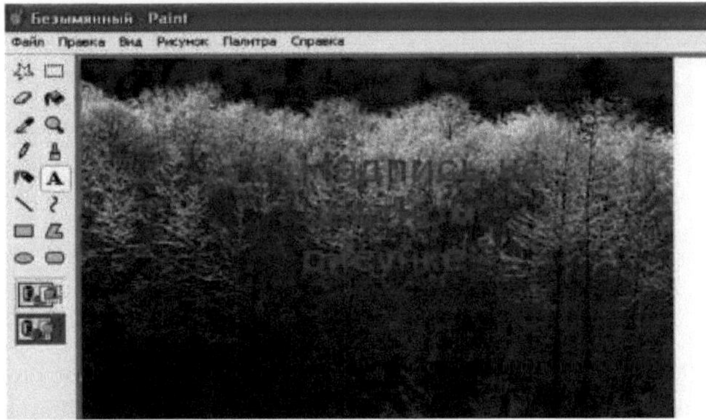

Fig. 3.13. Example of text input on a coloured drawing

Reporting Form:

When carrying out practical work, it is necessary to:

- Write down the number and topic of the class.
- Write down the assignment.
- Describe the performance of the work in detail.
- Answer the control questions.

Supervisory Questions:

1. What is the Control Panel for?

2. How do I change the Date and Time?
3. How can I change the Background, Screen Saver, Desktop Appearance?
4. What happens after activating the My Computer icon?
5. How can I copy the files and folders I need?
6. What methods of deleting files and folders do you know?
7. How can I change the mouse button assignment for left and right handed users?
8. How can I change the repeat rate of an input keyboard character?
9. How do you create a folder in your desired location on the disc?
10. How can you find the file you need?
11. What is the Paint programme used for?
12. How do I add a new colour to the colour palette?
13. How do you draw an accurate geometric figure?
14. How do I paste a picture from a file?
15. How do you make an inscription on a drawing?
16. How can a drawing be mirrored in the Paint programme?
17. **Recommended reading:** 1.1,1.2, 2.2.

Practical work No. 4

PLACEMENT, RETRIEVAL AND STORAGE OF INFORMATION. ANTI-VIRUS PROTECTION. FORMATTING FLOPPY DISCS. ARCHIVING FILES. WORKING WITH FLASH CARDS

Purpose of the lesson. Studying the technology of organisation of work with information in the Windows environment. Searching, saving information, checking for virus purity.

Formatting floppy discs. Archiving files. Learning how to work with flash cards.

Type of work: frontal

Lead time: 2 hours

Equipment: PC, floppy disk, flash card, Win Rar, Kaspersky Anti-Virus

The chronological map of the lesson is 80 minutes.

Organisational part: cleanliness of premises, equipment, sanitary and hygienic conditions.

Student attendance is 2 minutes.

Assessment of student knowledge: brief overview of the course, questions and answers with students - 10 minutes.

Setting a new theme - 20 minutes.

Determination and consolidation of the level of mastery of the subject - 35 minutes.

Test questions - 10 minutes.

Homework - 3 minutes.

Practical work requirements:

1. Answer the theoretical questions
2. Organise the tasks in a practical workbook

Theoretical material

Defragmentation is a program that combines fragmented files and folders on a computer disc, after which each file or folder in the volume occupies a single continuous space. As a result, files and folders are accessed more efficiently. By combining individual parts of files and folders, defragmentation software also combines free space on the disc into a single unit, making it less likely that new files will be fragmented.

When formatting is complete, a report of the formatting results will be displayed. If there are defective areas on the floppy disc, i.e. the total capacity of the disc does not match the available memory capacity, it is better not to use the floppy disc.

In Russia, antivirus problems have been professionally dealt with for many years mainly by two serious companies: Dialog Science (programs: Aidstest, Doctor WEB, ADinf, Sheriff complex) and Kaspersky Lab (Kami, AVP series programs).

Archiving files is the creation of a backup copy of files in case of unforeseen situations, and also in order to reduce the space occupied on the disc.

Assignment 4.1. Locating, searching and copying files/folders

Work order

1. In your folder, create three folders: "Copy", "Save", "Virus Check".
2. Find the calc.exe file corresponding to the "Calculator" program on the C: drive. To search, open the *Find* window from the Windows main menu *(Start/Find/Files and Folders),* on the *Name and Location* tab in the Name line enter the name of the file - calc.exe and select the area to search - the C: drive, including subfolders. Use the *Find* button to start the search.
3. Create a shortcut for the "Calculator" programme on the desktop. To do this, after finding the "calc.exe" file, drag its icon from the *Find* window to the workspace with the [Ctrl] key pressed.
4. Copy the calc.exe file to the Copy folder. To copy, place the cursor on the file and apply the *Edit/Copy* command. Open the *My Computer* window, then the C drive: My Documents, the group folder and your folder, the Copy folder. Then use the command *Edit/Paste.* The calc.exe file will be copied to the "Copy" folder.
5. Find files starting with ehr on all local hard drives *(Start/Find/Files and Folders).*On the *Name and Location* tab, in the Name line, type ehr* (Fig. 4.1). Select the area to search - local hard drives, including subfolders. An asterisk (*) in file and folder names replaces a group of random characters.

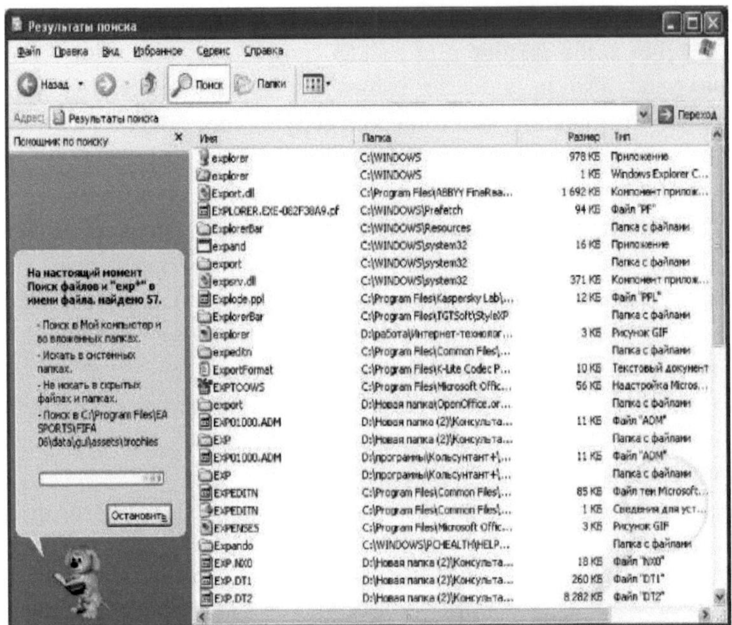

Fig. 4.1. Search for files starting with ehr

6. Sort files by name and select the group of files named explorer. To sort files and folders, set the *Find* window's tabular view *(View/Table).*

7. Open the "Explorer" programme and copy the selected files to the folder "Copy". To do this, select all files in the Search Results window using the Edit/Select All menu command. And copy the files.

8. Find all files modified in the past month *{Start/Find/Files and* Label"*/Date* tab*)* (Fig. 4.2). Record the number of found files in your workbook.

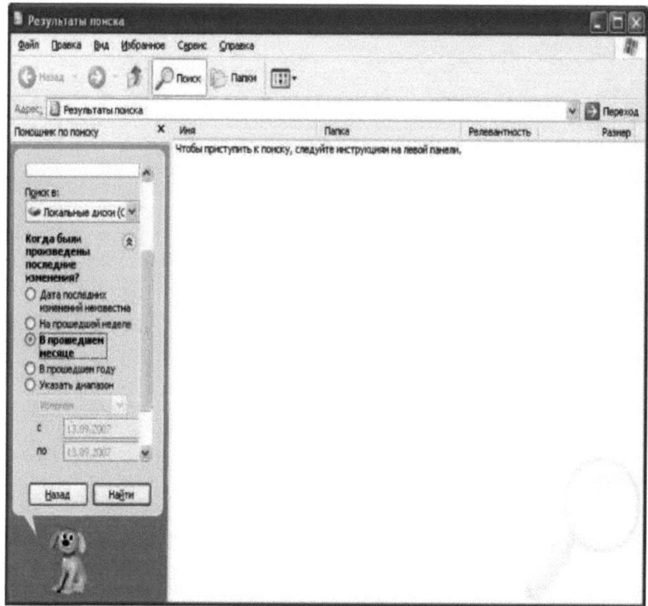

Fig.4.2 Search for files and folders modified during the last month

Task 4.2. Preparing floppy discs for work

Work order

To prepare a 3.5-inch (1.44 Mbyte) floppy drive for operation, you must format the floppy drive.

1. Insert the floppy disc into drive A:. Before formatting the floppy disc, make sure that the floppy disc write-protect window is closed.

2. Open the *My Computer* window.

3. Right-click on the *Disc 3.5* icon *(A:)* and select the *Format* command (Fig. 4.3).

Note. Be very careful when specifying a format object, because the formatting process partitions the disc and completely removes information from it.

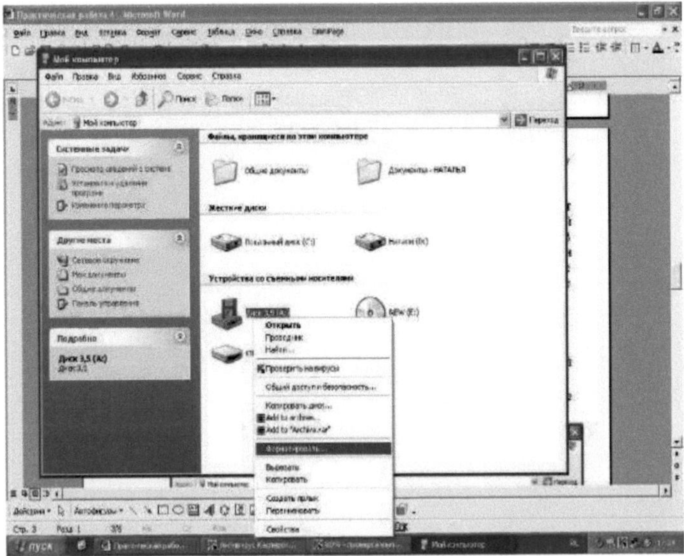
Fig. 4.3. Setting the floppy format command

4. Set the formatting options for the floppy drive *Quick* and click on the *Start* button.

5. If the floppy disc is slow to open, you should perform the following defragment the disc. To do this, right-click on the *Disk 3.5 (A)* icon and select *Properties/ Tools tab/ Perform defragmentation.* You can also perform an error check on the floppy disc.

Assignment 4.3. Work with flash-card to work

Work order

1. Insert the flash card into a connector on the system unit that is the right size (also called a USB connector).

2. Open My Computer and you will see that there is a new device - for example, KINGSTON (F:) (Fig.4.4).

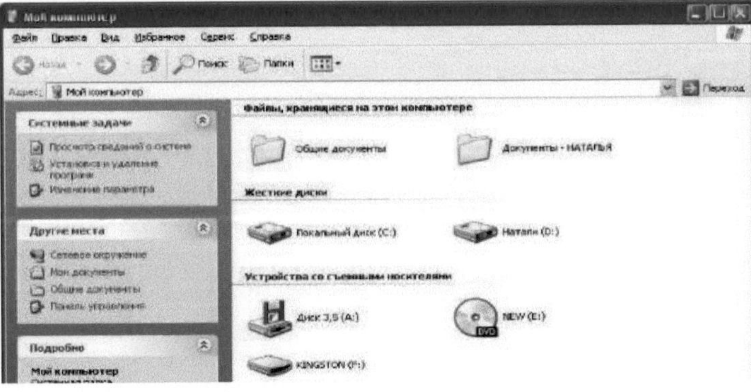

Fig. 4.4. My computer window

3. Check the capacity of the flash card. To do this, right-click on the flash card icon and select the *Properties* menu item.
4. Copy the folder with your last name in it and check how much space your folder takes up on the disc.
5. Delete your folder from the flash card.
6. Finish working with the flash card. To do this, right-click on the flash card icon on the taskbar and select the *Safely Remove Device* command in the menu that appears (Fig. 4.5). Then click Stop/ OK/ and close the window that informs that the device can be removed.

7. Remove the flash card from the slot.

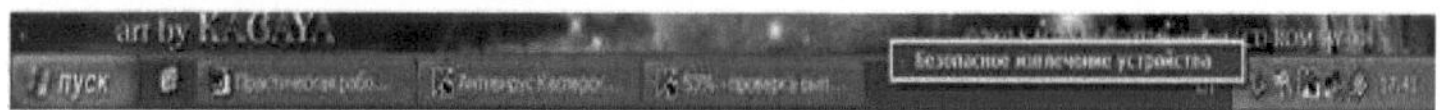

Figure 4.5. Safely remove the flash card device

Task 4.4. Saving files/folders

Work order

Open the electronic notepad (*Start/ Programs/ Standard/* Notepad). Type the text according to the sample in the notepad.

Sample text

The "Explorer" programme is designed to manage the Windows file system. "Explorer" displays the contents of folders, allows you to open, move, copy, delete, rename folders and files, run programs, display the tree of directories (folders). The right part of Explorer is an analogue of the My Computer window.

1. Save the typed text in the "Save" folder with the name "Sample Text" using the *File / Save* command (Fig. 4.6). In the "Folder" line specify the "Save" folder, in the "File name" line type the name "Sample text", and then click the Save button. The file will be saved on the C: disc in the "Save" folder.

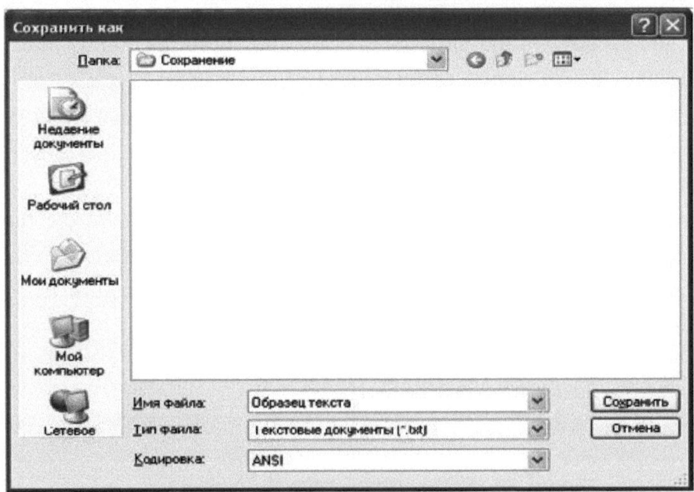

Fig. 4.6. File saving window

Task 4.5. Antivirus check of information on the C drive:

Work order

1. Run your existing antivirus programme,
e.g. Kaspersky AVP (Antiviral Toolkit Pro).
2. Specify the area to be checked - the C: drive (*Protection / Object Check / C-Drive - Check* (Fig. 4.7).

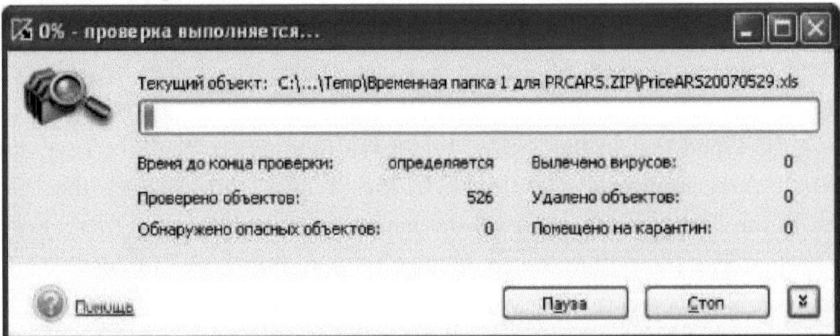

Fig. 4.7. Checking the C drive with antivirus software

3. Pay attention to the scanning process indicator. If the antivirus software detected viruses and cured the files (as shown in the scan report), run the C: drive scan process again and make sure that all viruses have been removed.
4. You can also check any objects such as Flash and floppy disks to ensure that you do not introduce viruses into your computer. Check the floppy disc for viruses and
cure them if you have them.

Task 4.6. Putting the files of your folder into an archive

Work order

1. Use My Documents to navigate to your folder.
2. To put the files of your folder into the archive do the following: right-click on the name of your folder, then select the Add to archive menu item, which means add to archive (Fig. 4.8).

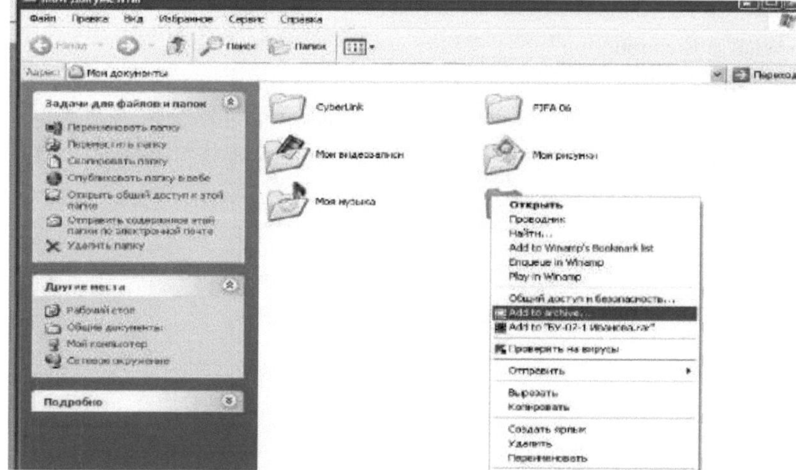

Fig. 4.8. Putting the required information into the archive

3. In the window that appears, select Compression method - Best. Click the OK button. An icon resembling several books will appear, this is the archive.
4. Extract files from the archive to the desktop. To do this, right-click on the file archive, in the window that appears select Extract Files, which means extract files, and specify the location - desktop.
5. Check it out, your folder should appear on your desktop.
6. Try to extract the files to the current folder. To do this, select the Extract Here menu item.

Reporting Form:

When carrying out practical work, it is necessary to:

- Write down the number and topic of the class.
- Write down the assignment.
- Describe the performance of the work in detail.
- Answer the control questions.

Supervisory Questions:

1. What is disc defragmentation?
2. What firms in Russia are engaged in anti-virus processes in the computer?
3. What is displayed on the screen after formatting is complete?
4. What happens during the formatting process?
5. How to find the required files if only the file name is known, but not known

expansion?

6. How do I finish working with the flash card?
7. How do I check My Computer for viruses?
8. How do I cure my computer of viruses?
9. How do I create a shortcut for the Calculator programme?
10. How do I save the file to the right place?
11. What is file archiving?
12. How do I archive the files I need?
13. How do I extract files from the archive to the current location?
14. How do I extract the files from the archive to the correct location?

Recommended reading: 1.1,1.2, 2.2.

Practical work No. 5

CREATING DOCUMENTS IN MS WORD. FONT FORMATTING

Purpose of the class. Study of information technology of creating, formatting and saving documents in MS WORD.

Type of work: frontal

Lead time: 2 hours

Equipment: PC, Microsoft Word

The chronological map of the lesson is 80 minutes.

Organisational part: cleanliness of premises, equipment, sanitary and hygienic conditions.

Student attendance is 2 minutes.

Assessing student learning: a brief overview of the subject,
Q&A with students - 10 minutes.

Setting a new theme - 20 minutes.

Determination and consolidation of the level of mastery of the subject - 35 minutes.

Test questions - 10 minutes.

Homework - 3 minutes.

Practical work requirements:

1. answer the theoretical questions
2. organise the tasks in the practical workbook

Theoretical material

Microsoft Word is a multifunctional word processing programme, a desktop publishing system.

A Microsoft Word document is a file with the extension .doc. To create a new document:

1. in the Microsoft Word programme window, select the File - New menu item.
2. In the Create Document dialogue box on the General tab, select the New Document object and click OK.

A pictographic menu is a row of icons consisting of fields of buttons with an image of one or another operation on them. In most cases, the buttons duplicate the most frequently used operations available in the regular menus.

A formatting panel is a row of icons consisting of elements required for text layout:

- *List fields* (they have a downward pointing arrow on the right side of the screen; clicking on the arrow opens a list window that lists the list items available for selection);
- *Pictogram fields* (if a text fragment is labelled, pressing some button on the

formatting ruler applies the function associated with this button).

Coordinate ruler - located above the document window. You can use the coordinate ruler to change paragraph indents, the length of the set line, and the width of columns.

Status bar - located on the bottom edge of the Word window. During data entry, this line displays information about the position of the input cursor, etc.

Text editing consists of deleting, adding, copying and transferring text fragments, spell checking using already known keyboard keys or pictographic menu.

The Standard and Formatting toolbars are opened automatically during standard installation of the programme. If they are closed and are not visible on the screen, you can open them from the *View* menu with *the Toolbars* command by ticking the checkbox in the list of toolbars.

If you select several symbols, you can keep the *Symbol* window open: successively select the symbols to be inserted with the mouse and click the Insert button.

A line of text is selected by single-clicking to the left of the line.

Task 5.1. Preparing to create a text document

Work order

1. Start the MS WORD text editor (Start / Programs / Microsoft office / Microsoft Word).
2. Set the programme parameters as shown in Fig. 5.1. (menu *Tools/* command *Parameters*, tab *View*).

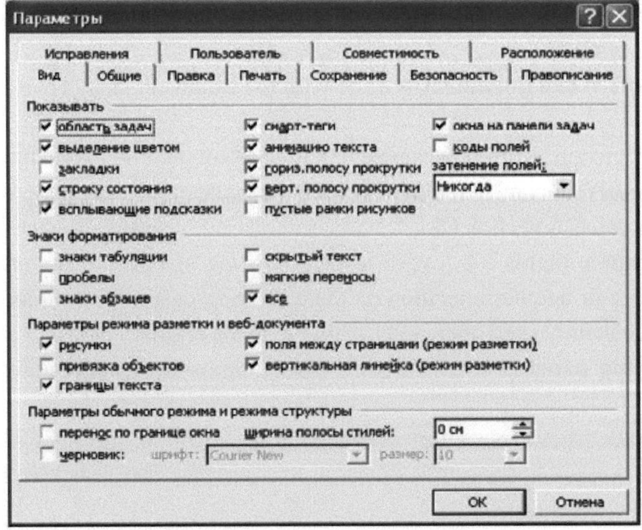

Fig. 5.1. Setting Microsoft Word parameters

3. Study the toolbar buttons *(Standard* and *Formatting)* of Microsoft Word (Fig. 5.2) by moving the mouse cursor to them.

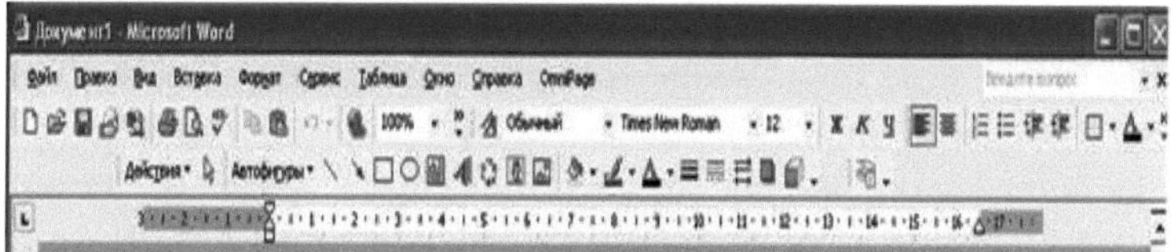

Fig. 5.2. Microsoft Word toolbars ("Standard" and "Formatting")

4. Set the screen view to *Normal* (menu *View,* command *Normal).* **Task 5. 2. Typing**

Work order

1. Type two paragraphs of text using the sample below (use the toolbar buttons to set the font type to Times New Roman, font size 14, italic). In the typed text, bold the names of menu items and commands.

Sample for recruitment

To visualise how text is arranged on the sheet, use the *Page Layout* view. To set this view, use the *View* menu and select *Page Layout.*

If you cannot see the edges of the document on the screen, select Scale to Width (*View* menu, *Scale to Width* command*).*

Task 5.3. Changing the screen view

Work order

1. Set the *Page Layout* mode - (*View/Page Layout* menu*).* Notice how the screen appearance has changed.
2. To select the optimal document size on the screen, set the below listed scale views *(View/Scale)* in the order listed *(Fig. 5*.3). Note how the screen view changes:

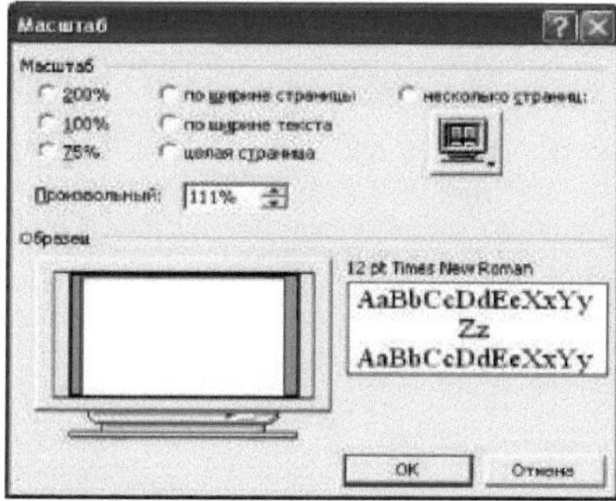

Figure 5. 3. Setting the scale

- standard 500% and 75%;
- random 38% and 130%;

- a few pages;
- page in its entirety;
- across the width of the page.

Leave the last set scale view "Width" for working with the document.

Task 5.4. Inserting symbols

Insert the following symbols after the text (*Insert* menu, *Symbol* command) (Figure 5.4).

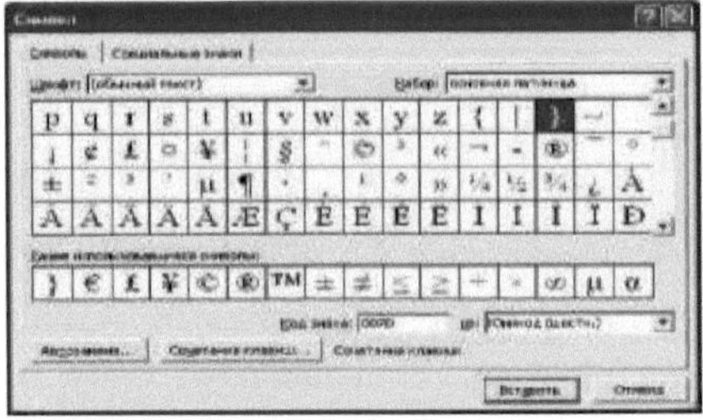

Fig.5.4 Inserting symbols into text

©, §, ® - tab *Special symbols;*

@, $, 3/4 - *Symbols* tab, font - plain text;

F, £, € - *Symbols* tab, font - plain text, set - *Money Symbols;*

|[J I Ol O) J J J[1] 'I - *Symbols* tab, font - Wingdings.

Note. If you do not see the desired symbols, you must select a different font type in the Font area of the *Symbol* window.

Task 5.5. Text formatting

Work order

1. Set different font sizes in the first paragraph of the typed text (by selecting words with the mouse or with the [Shift], [Ctrl] and -4 keys): the first word - 22 pt, the second -18 pt, the third - 14 pt, the fourth -10 pt. *{Format/Font/Font tab)* (Figure 5. 5).
2. *Format* every two words in the second paragraph on the first line in a different colour *(Format/Font/Font tab.*

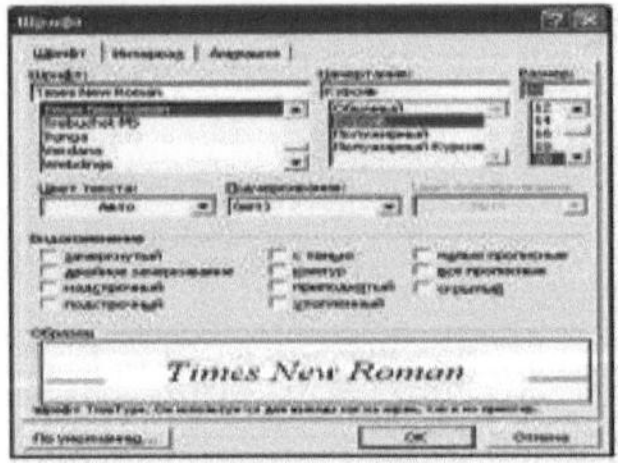

Fig. 5.5. Setting font parameters

3. Make the following transformations in the second paragraph, highlighting

the desired words *(Format/Font/Font tab):*

The first two words are in **bold; the** second two words are **in bold; the** second two words are **in**

- *in italics; the* third two words are underlined:

the next two words *in italics* + **bold** + underline.

4. Set different types of underlines in the first paragraph *(Format/Font/Font tab):*

the first word with a single underline,

second - with a dotted underline, third - with a double underline.

5. Type the word "effect". Copy it five times *(Edit/Copy, Edit/Paste)* and apply the following modifications *(Format/Font/Font* tab*):*

~~Effect~~ (crossed out);

Effect (upper index or superscript);

Effect (lowercase or subscript);

EFFECT (small caps);

E^FSHGIH uppercase + outline + bold).

Brief Synopsis. Text copying consists of four operations:

- Select a text (or a fragment) to copy;
- writing the fragment to the memory buffer *(Edit/Copy);*
- setting the cursor to the place where the fragment to be copied is called;
- call from the memory buffer *(Edit/Paste).*

6. Apply the Fireworks animation effect to the first page of the first paragraph *(Format/Font, Animation* tab*).*

7. In the source text on the words "Page Layout" set the spacing to 10 pt. *(Format/Font* /Interval *tab/sparse* spacing by 10 pt.) (Fig. 5.6).

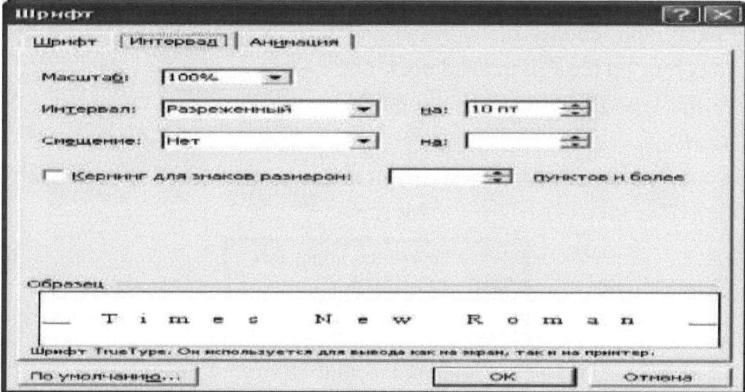

Figure 5.6. Setting the sparse text view

8. On the words "Width Scale", set a wavy underline and blue font colour.

9. Highlight the second paragraph of text and change the font type to Arial. Notice the change in the appearance of the font.

Task 5.6. Text framing and filling

Work order

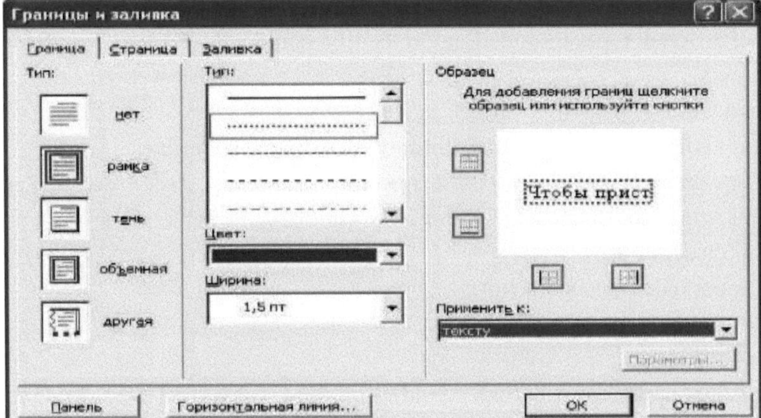

Figure 5. 7. Framing text with a frame

1. Frame the first line of the text. To do this, select the first line line, select the *Borders and Fill* command in the *Format* menu, set the line colour - blue, thickness - 1.5 pt, line type - solid line; apply - to text, border type - frame on the *Borders* tab (Figure 5.7).

If you apply the frame "to text", the frame will border only the selected words, and if you apply the frame "to paragraph", the frame will take the size of the sheet width without taking into account the margins.

2. Fill the second paragraph of the text with colour. To do this, select the second paragraph, choose the *Borders and Fill* command in the *Format* menu, choose a colour on the *Fill* tab and click *OK.*

3. Save the typed document in your folder with the name "Ivanova 1.doc" { *File/Save As...*).

Create your business card enclosed in a frame:

Moscow,

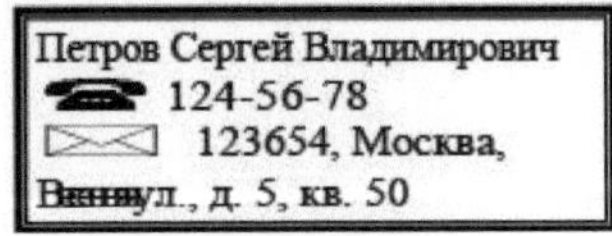

Vsnyaul. 5, flat 50.

Additional task

Task 5.7.

Using all the techniques you know about creating, copying and formatting text documents, complete the assignment in MS Word following the sample, trying to create a document as close as possible to the original assignment in terms of appearance.

|Format - Font|

|Format - Borders and Fill|

Computer technology

Computer technology

Computer technology

Computer technology

Computer technology

Computer ~~technology~~

Computer technology

Computer^{техн} ologies

^{Компью}терные ^{техн}ологии

~~Компьютерные~~ технологии

COMPUTER TECHNOLOGY

Computer technology||

Reporting Form:

When carrying out practical work, it is necessary to:

- Write down the number and topic of the class.
- Write down the assignment.
- Describe the performance of the work in detail.
- Answer the control questions.

Supervisory Questions:

1. What is Microsoft Word?
2. What is the Pictorial Menu?
3. What is the purpose of the Format Panel?
4. What is a Coordinate Ruler?
5. Where is the status bar, what does it display?
6. How do I enable the standard panel and formatting panel?
7. Do you have to close the Character window if you want to insert multiple characters at the same time?
8. How can you select a line of text?
9. How do I start a Microsoft Word programme?
10. How do I put text in a frame?
11. How do I fill text with a specific colour?

Recommended reading: 1.1,1.2, 2.2.

Practical work No. 6

DESIGN OF PARAGRAPHS IN DOCUMENTS. COLONTITULES

Purpose of the lesson. Studying the information technology of creating and formatting text paragraphs in MS Word.

Type of work: frontal

Lead time: 2 hours

Equipment: PC, Microsoft Word

The chronological map of the lesson is 80 minutes.

Organisational part: cleanliness of premises, equipment, sanitary and hygienic conditions.

Student attendance is 2 minutes.

Assessment of students' knowledge : brief overview of the subject, questions and answers with students -10 minutes.

Setting a new theme - 20 minutes.

Determination and consolidation of the level of mastery of the subject -35 minutes.

Test questions - 10 minutes.

Homework - 3 minutes.

Practical work requirements:

1. Answer the theoretical questions
2. Organise the tasks in the practical workbook

Theoretical material

When typing on the keyboard, the words in a sentence are automatically moved to the next line. **A paragraph** in a text document is a part of text located between two consecutive presses of the Enter key.

Each paragraph has the following parameters that determine the arrangement of characters in the paragraph:

- levelling;
- level;
- indentation;
- interval;
- tabulation.

In addition, there are a number of parameters that determine the position of a paragraph on the page in relation to the preceding and following paragraphs:

- banning dangling strings;
- not to break a paragraph;
- don't pull away from the next one;
- from a new page;
- prohibition of line numbering;

- prohibition of automatic word transfer.

All these parameters are set as desired by the user and are defined by default in document templates according to predefined styles.

Paragraph settings can be set before typing or changed while editing text using the **Format - Paragraph** menu item.

Alignment is the method by which the beginnings and endings of lines are set relative to each other.

A paragraph of text is **selected** by double-clicking to the left of the paragraph.

Paragraph framing is the process of putting a **paragraph** in a frame.

A **footer** is any design that repeats at the top or bottom of each page. Date, time and page numbers are set using the Columns panel buttons. Switching to the footer is also done with the button in the Columns panel. Footers are visible only in the Page Layout view.

Task 6.1. Formatting text paragraphs

Work order

1. Launch the Microsoft Word text editor.
2. Set font parameters: font typeface - Times New Roman, font size - 14, font size - normal.
3. Type one paragraph of text based on the sample.

Sample text

Before typing the text it is necessary to set paragraph parameters in addition to font parameters. To do this, use the Format/Absetup command and in the opened window set the parameters of text alignment on the sheet of paper, parameters of the first line, line spacing and spacing.

4. Copy the typed paragraph of text five times (Edit/Copy, Edit/Paste).
5. Having selected the first paragraph of the text, set the following paragraph parameters (Format/Abstract/Abstract/Spacing tab) (Fig. 6. 1):

first line - standard indentation;
line spacing - one and a half lines; alignment - width.

6. With the third paragraph of text selected, set the following paragraph options:

first line - standard indentation;
line spacing - single line;
alignment - left edge.

7. With the fifth paragraph of the text highlighted , set the following paras paragraph metres:

first line - none; line spacing - no line spacing
double; alignment - to the right edge.

8. With the sixth paragraph of text selected, set the following paragraph

options:
first line - indent by 2.5 cm;
line spacing - multiplier 1.3;
выравнивание — по центру.

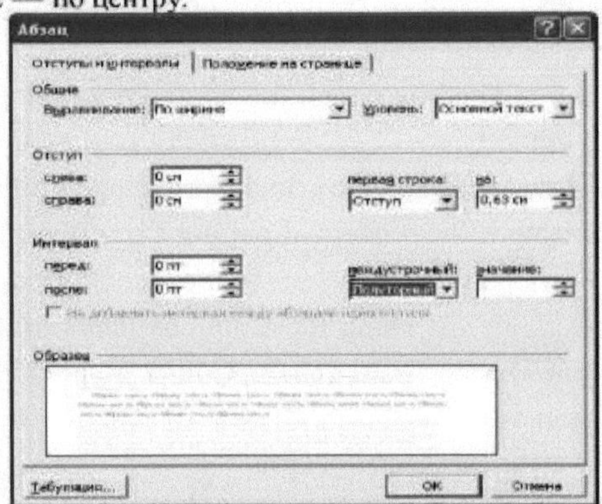

Рис. 6.1. Задание параметров абзаца текста

9. Having selected the second paragraph of the text, set the following paragraph parameters: first line - indent by 1.5 cm;

right indent -4 cm;
line spacing - multiplier 1.8;
alignment - width.

10. Having selected the fourth paragraph of the text, set the following paragraph parameters: first line - indent by 2 cm;
indentation on the right -3 cm;
indentation on the left -6 cm;
line spacing - multiplier 2.5;
alignment - width.

Task 6.2. Framing paragraphs

Work order

When selecting paragraphs of text, set the following frame options (Format/Borders and Fill/Border tab).
First paragraph:
line type - normal line;
colour - auto;
width - 0.5 pt;
apply to a paragraph;
type of framing - frame.
Third paragraph (Figure 6.2):
line type - normal line;

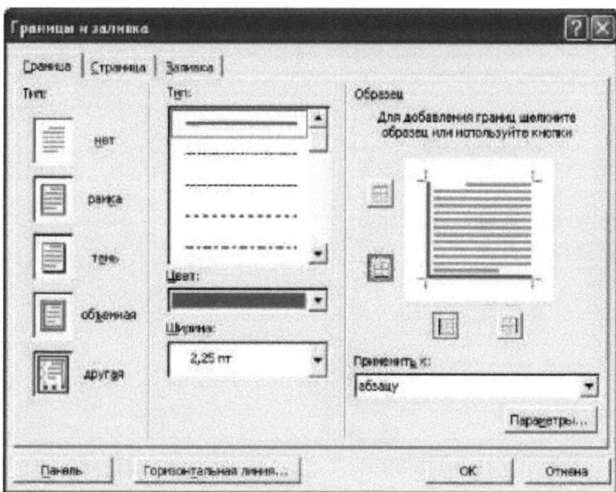

Fig. 6.2. Setting parameters of text borders (frame)

colour blue;
width - 2.25 pts;
apply to a paragraph;
type of framing - lines on the left and bottom.
Fifth paragraph:
line type - dotted line;
the colour is red;
width - 1.5 pt;
apply to a paragraph;
type of framing - lines on the left and right.

Assignment 6. 3. Filling paragraphs

Work order

When selecting paragraphs of text, set the following fill options (Format/Borders and Fill/Fill tab) (Fig.6. 3).
Second paragraph:
fill - light yellow colour;
pattern - 10%;
apply to a paragraph.
Fourth paragraph:
fill - light blue colour;
pattern, no;
apply it to the text.
Sixth paragraph:
the fill is a lilac colour;
pattern - light diagonally downwards; apply - to paragraph.

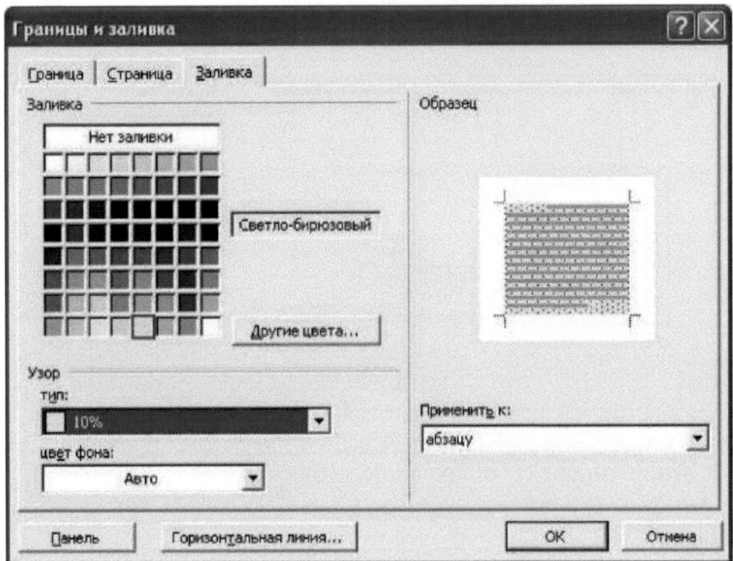

Fig. 6..3. Setting the paragraph filler

Task 6.4. Setting inter-paragraph spacing Work order

Select all the text with the Edit/Select All command and set the spacing between paragraphs to 24 pts. with the Format/Abstance command/Integration tab/Interval before - 24 pts.

Task 6.5. Setting footers

Work order

1. Set the document view to Page Layout (View/Page Layout).
2. Set the document footer (View/Columns) (Fig. 6.4). Learn the purpose of the Columns panel buttons by moving the mouse cursor to them. Enter the following information in the footers:

in the header - full name, date, time;

in the footer - the name of the educational institution and page numbers.

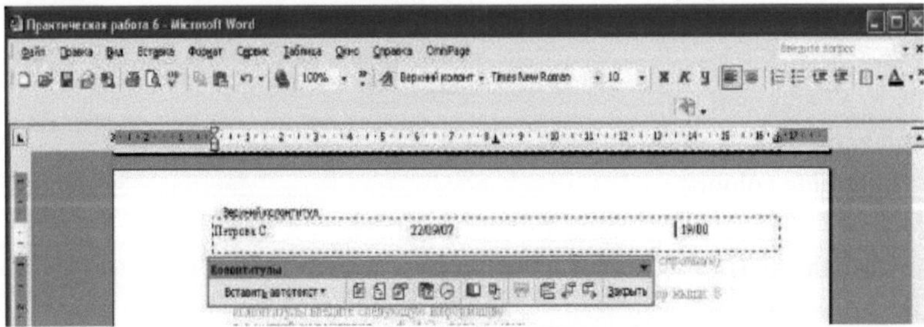

Figure 6. 4. Setting the header

Header/Footer. Please note that when you enter footers, the main text becomes pale in colour and inaccessible. You can end work with footers by pressing the Close button of the Columns panel.

3. Set the page parameters and the distance from the edge to the footer as in fig. 6.5. (File/Page Options).

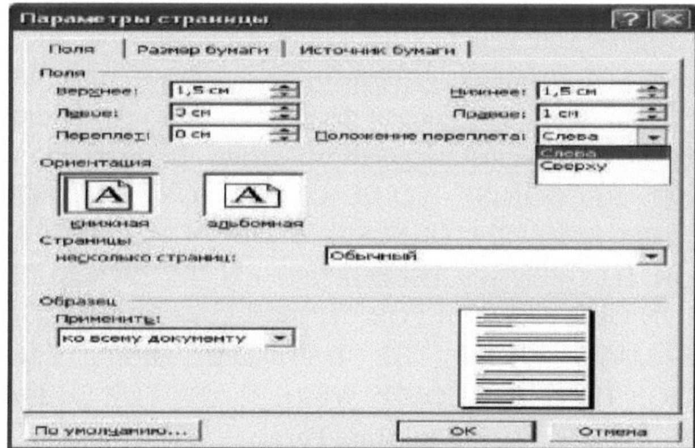

Figure 6.5. Setting page parameters and distance from the edge to the footer

4. Change the screen view to normal (View/Ordinary). Note that footers are not visible in the normal document view.

.5. Save the typed document in your folder with the name "iv;puv;12.c1os".

Additional task

Task 6.6. Using copying and formatting, type according to the sample:

We cannot recognise your claim for the following reason. According to clause 6 of our contract, you undertook to open by telegraph an irrevocable letter of credit in our favour for the full value of the goods within 5 days from the date of our telegraphic notification that the goods were ready for shipment.

We cannot recognise your claim for the following reason. According to clause 6 of our contract, you undertook to open by telegraph an irrevocable letter of credit in our favour for the full value of the goods within 5 days from the date of our telegraphic notification that the goods were ready for shipment.

We cannot recognise your claim for the following reason. According to clause 6 I of our contract, you undertook to open by telegraph an irrevocable letter of credit in

I our favour for the full value of the goods within 5 days from the date of our I
I telegraphic notification that the goods are ready for shipment.i

We cannot recognise your claim for the following reason. According to clause 6 of our contract, you undertook to open by telegraph an irrevocable letter of credit in our favour for the full value of the goods within 5 days from the date of our telegraphic notification that the goods were ready for shipment.

<u>We cannot recognise your claim for the following reason. According to clause 6 of our contract, you undertook to open by telegraph an irrevocable letter of credit in our favour for the full value of the goods within 5 days from the date of our</u> telegraphic notification that the goods were ready for shipment.

We cannot recognise your claim for the following reason. According to clause 6 of our contract, you undertook to open by telegraph an irrevocable letter of credit in <u>our favour for the full</u> value of the goods within 5 days from the date of our <u>telegraphic</u> notification that the goods were ready for shipment.

WE CANNOT RECOGNISE YOUR CLAIM FOR THE FOLLOWING REASON. PURSUANT TO CLAUSE. 6 OF OUR CONTRACT, YOU UNDERTOOK TO OPEN BY TELEGRAPH AN IRREVOCABLE LETTER OF CREDIT IN OUR FAVOUR FOR THE FULL VALUE OF THE GOODS WITHIN 5 DAYS FROM THE DATE OF OUR TELEGRAPHIC NOTIFICATION THAT THE GOODS WERE READY FOR SHIPMENT.

Reporting Form:

When carrying out practical work, it is necessary to:

- Write down the number and topic of the class.
- Write down the assignment.
- Describe the performance of the work in detail.
- Answer the control questions.

Supervisory Questions:

1. How do I set the paragraph parameters?
2. How do I copy the text I want?
3. How to set indents, indents for a paragraph?
4. What do you need to do to frame, fill paragraphs?
5. How do I set the spacing between paragraphs?
6. What do I need to do to insert footers into a document?

Recommended reading: 1.1,1.2, 2.2.

Practical work No. 7

CREATING AND FORMATTING TABLES IN MS WORD

Class Objective. Study of information technology of creating and formatting tables in MS Word.

Type of work: frontal

Lead time: 2 hours

Equipment: PC, Microsoft Word

The chronological map of the lesson is 80 minutes.

Organisational part: cleanliness of premises, equipment, sanitary and hygienic conditions.

Student attendance is 2 minutes.

Assessing student learning: a brief overview of the subject,
Q&A with students - 10 minutes.

Setting a new theme - 20 minutes.

Determination and consolidation of the level of mastery of the subject - 35 minutes.

Test questions - 10 minutes.

Homework - 3 minutes.

Practical work requirements:

1. answer the theoretical questions
2. organise the tasks in the practical workbook

Theoretical material

Tables are often used to arrange ordered text, numeric and graphic elements in a document. A table is also convenient to use for other design options, for example, for placing text in several columns.

A **table** consists of horizontal **rows** and vertical **columns**, the intersection of which forms a **cell.** You can change the size of cells using table properties. To do this, just place the cursor inside the table, select the Table Properties command in the Table menu (Fig. 7.3). In the appeared dialogue window on the Table tab you can change the size, alignment, fairing. On the Row tab you can change the height of rows, and on the Column tab - the width of columns, on the Cell tab - the cell size.

To sort the data in the columns of a table, select the text fragment you want to sort.

To merge or split cells, select a group of cells and apply the Table/Merge-Split Cells command. To change the width of a single cell, select the cell, then change the cell width.

It is easy to apply formulas, different background filling to table elements, automatic repetition of header (header) on each page is possible.

Task 7.1. Creating and formatting a table

Work order

1. Launch the Microsoft Word text editor.
2. Set page parameters (A4 paper size, portrait orientation; margins: left -3 cm, right -2 cm; top -3 cm; bottom -2.5 cm) using the File/Page Parameters command.
3. Set the paragraph format (first line - indented, line spacing - one and a half).
4. Create a 2x9 table using the Table/ Insert/Table command (Fig. 7.1) or the Add Table button from the toolbar by clicking and advancing the table with the left mouse button (Fig. 7.2).
5. Change the width of the columns according to the sample Table 1:

point the mouse arrow at the vertical table separator, the mouse arrow will look like a separator;

by clicking and advancing the separator with the left mouse button, set the desired width of the table columns.

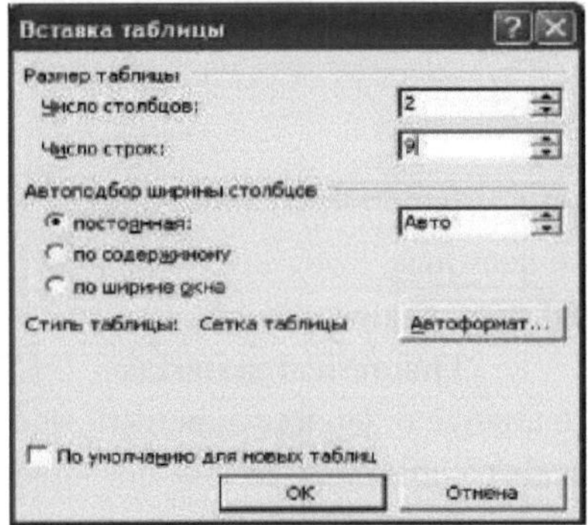

Fig.7.1. Setting table parameters from the Tables menu

The table parameters can be auto-selected using the Table/AutoSelect menu command. Microsoft Word will automatically select the width, columns or rows depending on the width of the sheet and the amount of text in each cell.

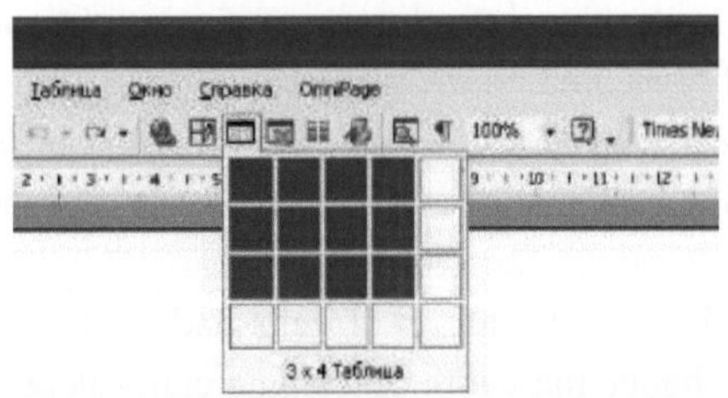

Fig. 7.2. Setting a table from the toolbar

6. Highlight the first line of the table (header) and set the paragraph alignment type to centre.

7. Highlight the second column of the table and set the paragraph alignment type to centre.
8. Fill in the table by moving around the table using the [Tab], [Shift+Tab] keys.
9. Add a new row to the table by placing the cursor in the right cell of the bottom row of the table and press the [Tab] key or use the Table/Add/Add/Row Above/Below command, having previously placed the cursor in any cell of the bottom row of the table.
10. Select the entire table by placing the cursor in any cell of the table and executing the Table/Select/Table command or clicking the left mouse button on the cross-shaped mouse pointer in the upper left corner of the table behind its outline.

Table 1

Monetary parameters	Amount, USD billion
Overnight loans and other	17
One-day repurchase agreements	64
Cash	232
Money market mutual funds	318
Savings deposits	410
Money market deposit accounts	485
T ransaction deposits These include: demand deposits other	563 277 286
Total: M 1	795
Term deposits	1143
Total: M 2	3232

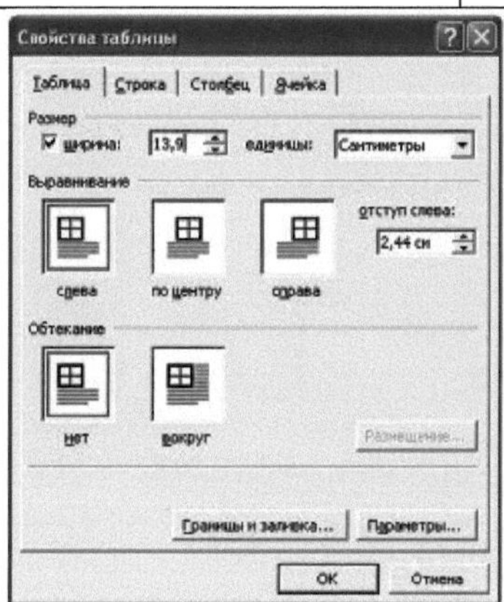

Fig. 7.3. Table property window

11. Frame the table according to the sample using the Format/Borders and Fill command.

12. Sort (in ascending order) the data of the second column of the table, highlighted by the bold line.

Select the Sort command from the Table menu (Figure 7. 4). In the Text sorting window that opens, use the list to select whether you want to sort the whole paragraphs or only the text typed before the tab character. In the Type list, select the desired sorting method - as text, number or date. Use the ascending and descending selection buttons to select the desired method. Click the OK button.

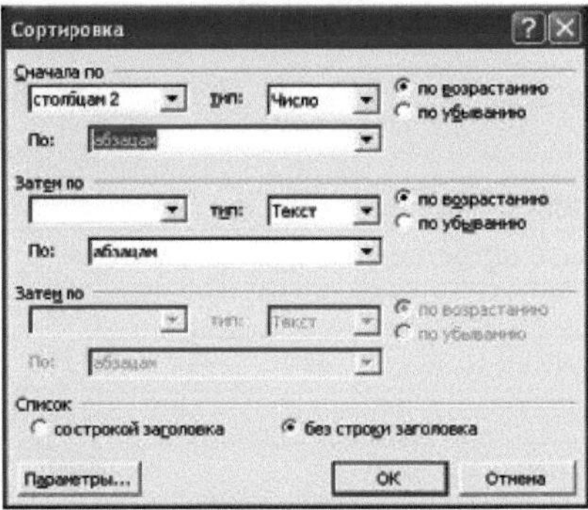

Figure 7.4. Sorting data in the table

13. Save the file in your folder with the name "Table 1".

14. Autoformat the table. To do this, place the cursor inside the table, select the AutoFormat and Table Format - Table Columns 1 command in the Table menu (Figure 7.5).

15. Save the formatted table in your folder with the name "Table 2" (File/Save As).

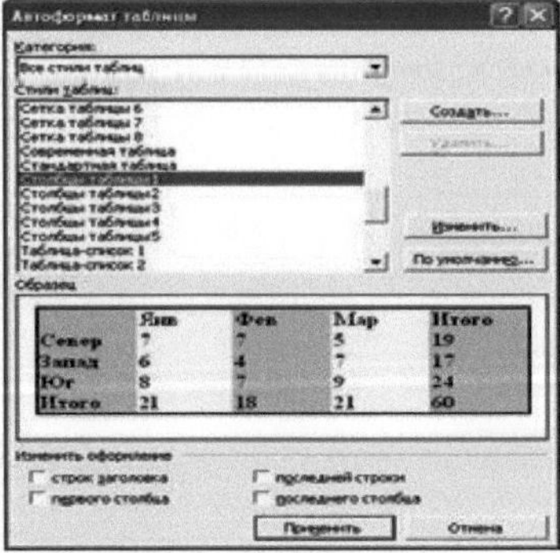

Fig.7.5 Setting the table AutoFormat

Additional tasks

Task 7.2. Type tables in MS Word according to the sample (Tables 2-3)

Table 2

Date	Turnover		Revenue	Sections			Composition	Total
	Plan	Fact		1	2	3		
1999	13 542	13457	4578632	4 562	1547	1247	25	1247
2000	16 754	15 486	5 789 642	7852	1255	2525	45	1554
2001	13 658	14358	1257896	1554	1236	6 457	76	15 577
2002	56 783	58762	125 584	2 336	1255	2155	89	12 544

T"Table 3

Task 7.3. Type a table in MS Word according to the following sample

HP O printer/scanner/copier ffisJet R65

Technical specifications				Ordering information	
	HP PhotoREt 11 technology with 600x600 multilayer colour overlay: black with HP Colour Enhancement Technology (KYt) 600x600; colour with HP PhotoREt 11' technology			All-in-one printer/scanner/copier	
				C6693A	HP OffisJet R65
				C6692A	HP OffisJet R45
Print	Printing method	Thermal on demand inkjet printing		Cables	
	Printer control language	P PC Level 3 or PCL3GU1		C2946A	IEEE I235A-C parallel cable, Zm
	Load	3000 pages per month (average)		C2947A	IEEE 1235A-C Parallel Cable, 10 m
	Print speed (s/min)	Black	Coloured	Inkjet printer cartridges	
	Fast Ordinary	11 5,1	8,5 3,6	51645A	Large black HP cartridge
	Best	4,4		C1876G	Colour cartridge
				C1879D	Large HP triple-colour colour cartridge
				54389G	Black cartridge

	Printer resolution	Black	Coloured	
	Fast Normal Best	600x300 600x300 600x600	300x300 600 x 600 600 x 600	
	Built-in fonts	Courier, Courier Italic; CG Times, CG Times Italic; Letter Gothic, Letter Gothic		

Reporting Form:

When carrying out practical work, it is necessary to:

- Write down the number and topic of the class.
- Write down the assignment.
- Describe the performance of the work in detail.
- Answer the control questions.

Supervisory Questions:

1. Give the definition of a table.
2. What is a cell?
3. What ways of creating tables do you know?
4. How do I sort the data within a table?
5. How to set the Autoformat of a table?
6. How do I set the table borders and fill?

Recommended reading: 1.1,1.2, 2.2.

Practical work No. 8

CREATING LISTS IN TEXT DOCUMENTS. RINGS. BOOK. FORMATTING REGISTERS. OBJECT INSERTION IN DOCUMENT. PRINT PREPARATION

Purpose of the lesson. Studying the information technology of creating lists in MS Word, creating text with columns, text design, inserting objects into the text in MS Word.

Type of work: frontal

Lead time: 2 hours

Equipment: PC, Microsoft Word, printer

The chronological map of the lesson is 80 minutes.

Organisational part: cleanliness of premises, equipment, sanitary and hygienic conditions.

Student attendance is 2 minutes.

Assessing student learning: a brief overview of the subject,
Q&A with students - 10 minutes.

Setting a new theme - 20 minutes.

Determination and consolidation of the level of mastery of the subject - 35 minutes.

Test questions - 10 minutes.

Homework - 3 minutes.

Practical work requirements:

1. Answer the theoretical questions
2. Organise the tasks in a practical workbook

Theoretical material

You can organise three types of lists in **Microsoft Word** documents:

- **numbered** - at the beginning of each paragraph its number from the list is set. Arabic and Roman numerals, symbols of the Latin alphabet and some compound expressions, e.g. first, second, etc., can be used as a number;
- **labelled** - some marker is placed at the beginning of each paragraph, e.g. -, -, etc.;
- **multi-level** - at the beginning of each paragraph, depending on its level in the list, both a marker and a number can be set.

When creating lists, you can use two methods: you can set list options while you are typing, or you can apply a list view after you have typed.

When working with a multilevel list, you should select the *Multilevel* list type and then use the toolbar buttons that allow you to assign the appropriate level to the selected list items.

To change the type of markers by levels, in the *List* window after selecting the labelled list click the *Change* button (Fig. 8.3). In the opened window *Change multilevel list* set the list level and select the marker type for this level (in the *Numbering zone).* If you are not satisfied with the marker type in the *Numbering* zone, select the *New marker* command in the same zone, and the symbol table will open.

To add a letter, place the cursor on the first line of text and then select *Format/letter.*

If you want to insert a picture into the text, you need to select the Insert - Picture - Pictures menu item.

To insert autofigures, select the *Insert/Drawing/Autofigures* menu item.

To resize a drawing, activate it (by clicking on the drawing) and move the drawing marker to a new location.

You can move a drawing around the document by dragging it with the mouse.

Page options include page size, margins (distance from page edge to text), distance from page edge to footer, and page orientation. The page options are set using the *File/Page* Options command*, the Margins* and *Paper Size* tabs.

Task 8.1. Creating lists

First method: setting the list parameters as you type.

Sample text with a numbered list

Elementary operations of the information process include: collection,
Transforming information, inputting it into a computer; transferring information; storing and processing information; providing information to the user.

Work order

1. Launch the Microsoft Word text editor.
2. Type the first line of the sample text, press [Enter].
3. Click the *Numbering* button in the toolbar*, the* number 1 will appear (if you click the *Marker* button, the first marker will appear in the row).
4. Type the text of the first item and press [Enter]. The entry point moves to the next line, which is immediately given a sequential number (2, 3, etc.), or a new marker mark appears.
5. To terminate the list on the next page, click the *Numbering* (or *Marker)* button again to remove the corresponding list item from the row.
6. Convert an already prepared list from a numbered list to a labelled list. To do this, select all items in the list (as a set of lines) and press the button *Marker*. Notice how the appearance of the list has changed.

The second method: overlaying list options after typing.

1. Type the text using the sample below.

1.1.6 lines (future list items) enter as separate paragraphs by pressing [Enter| at the end of each line.

Sample text

Elementary operations of the information process include:
collecting, transforming information, inputting it into a computer;
transferring information;
storage and processing of information;
providing information to the user.

2. Copy the typed text fragment four times *(Edit/Copy, Edit/Paste).*
3. Create a single-level numbered list. To do this

select the list part of the first fragment (3...6 lines), set the *Format/List* command, select the *Numbered* tab and choose the usual numbering type, then click *OK* (Fig. 8.1).

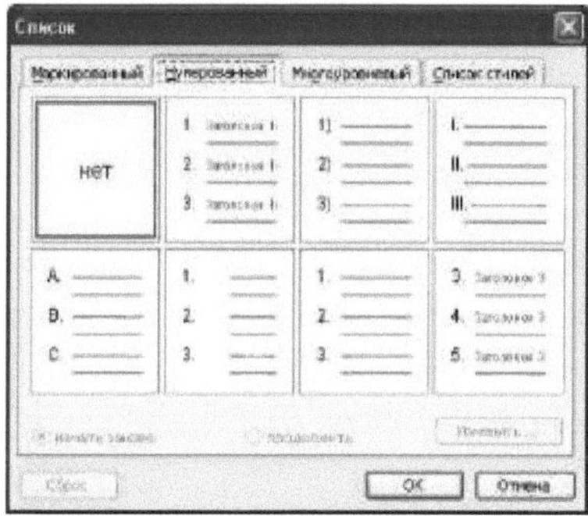

Fig. 8.1. Defining a single-level numbered list

4. Select the list part of the second fragment (3...6 lines) and form a single-level labelled list.

To do this, use theFormat/List command, select
Marked tab and set the list marker view.

5. Select the list part of the third fragment (3...6 lines) and form a multi-level numbered list.

To do this, use theFormat/List command, select
Select the *Multilevel* tab and select the multilevel numbered list view. The numbering in the first level will be performed
list. To see the numbering of the second, third, etc. levels, you need to increase the indentation using the button on the toolbar *Increase indentation.*

6. Select the list part of the fourth fragment (3...6 lines) and form a multi-level labelled list. To do this, use the *Format/List* command, select
tab *Multilevel* and the multi-level labelled list view (Fig. 8.2).

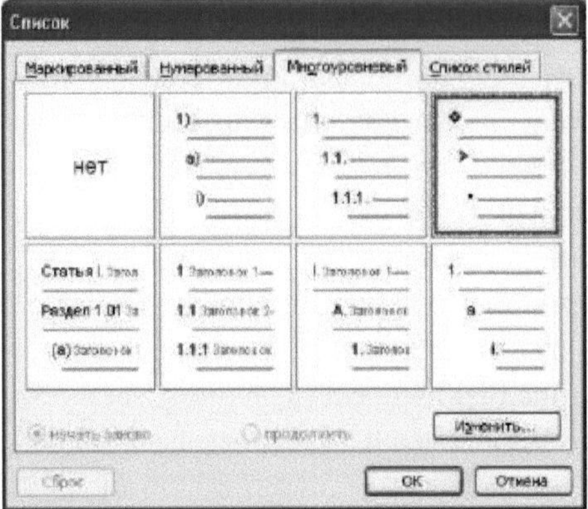

Fig.8.2 Define a multi-level labelled list Select a new type of marker and click *OK*.

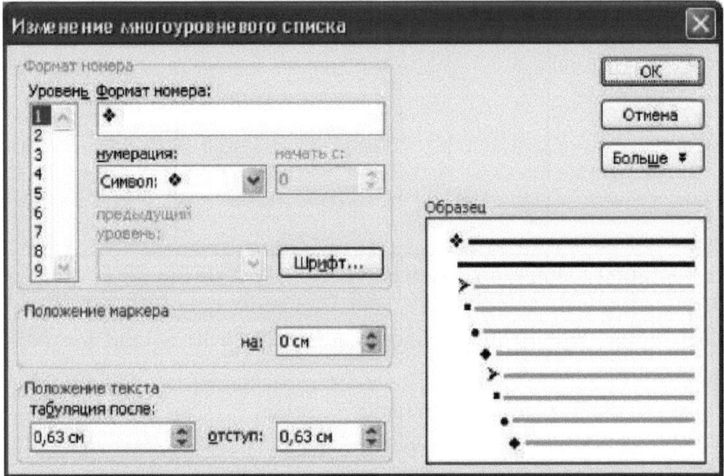

Fig.8.3. Changing markers of a multilevel list

Numbering by markers in the first level of the list will take place. To see the numbering by markers of the second, third, etc. levels, it is necessary to increase the indentation using the *Increase indentation* toolbar button.

7. Save the document in your folder with the name "Document 3" *(File/Save As)*.

Additional tasks

Task 8.2. Type lists (single-level and multi-level) in MS Word according to the following samples

Work order

Copying text by dragging and dropping

1 Identify the text to be copied and its location

Appointments.
2. Select the text and drag it with the mouse button pressed to a new location. Release the mouse button where the copied fragment should appear.
3. Select *Copy* from the drop-down menu.

Copying text by dragging and dropping

> Identify the text to be copied and its destination.

> Highlight the text and drag it with *the* mouse button depressed to the new location. Release the mouse button where the copied fragment should appear.

> Select *Copy* from the drop-down menu.

Copying text by dragging and dropping

Identify the text to be copied and its destination.
Select the text and drag it while holding down the mouse button to a new location. Release the mouse button where you want the copied fragment to appear.
~~IB I 0~~|Select the item from the pop-up menu.
Copy.

Copying text by dragging and dropping

---

a) Identify the text to be copied and its destination.
b) Highlight a textile and drag it while holding down the button . to the new location. Release the mouse button where the copied fragment should appear.
c) From the drop-down menu, select *Copy*

Copying text by dragging and dropping

A. Identify the text to be copied and its destination.
B. Select the text and drag it while holding down the mouse button to a new location.
Release the mouse button where the fragment to be copied should appear.
| C. Select *Copy* from the drop-down menu.

Task 8.3. Creating multi-column documents Work order

1. Launch the Microsoft Word text editor.
2. Type one paragraph of text using the sample below (use the buttons on the toolbar to set the font type to Times New Roman and font size to 14).

Sample for recruitment

If you want to create columns like newspaper columns, or columns like those used in newsletters and brochures, you need to set Word to format your text accordingly. You can have multiple columns for the whole text of a document or just a selected part of it. It is best to type the text of a document before dividing it into multiple columns.

3. Copy the typed text fragment twice *(Edit/Copy, Edit/Paste).*

4. Highlight the first fragment and split it into two columns with a separator *(Format/Columns)* (Fig. 8.4).

5. Highlight the second piece of text and break it into three parts columns (*Format/Columns).*

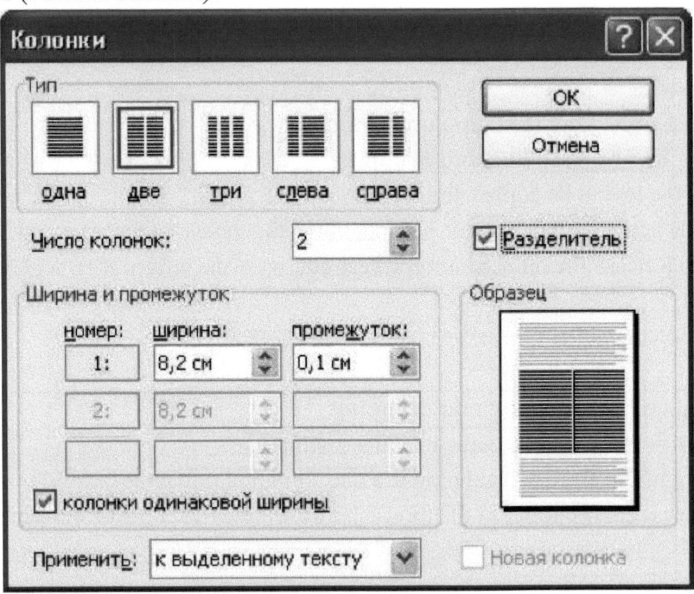

Figure 8.4. Breaking text into columns

Task 8.4. Formalisation of documents in alphabets

Work order

1. Insert the Primer into the text.
2. Set the parameters: height in lines - 2 cm, distance from text - 0.5 cm (Fig. 8.5).

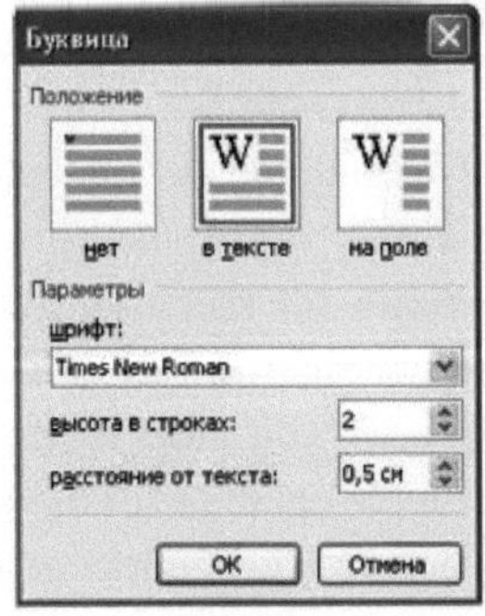

Figure 8.5. Setting the alphabet

Task 8.5. Changing the font case and text direction

Work order

1. By selecting individual lines of the third text fragment and using the command
Format/Register (Fig.8.6), format the text as follows:
the first line is "All caps."
the second line is "All lowercase."
third line, "Start with uppercase."
the fourth line is "Change Register";
line five is "As in sentences."

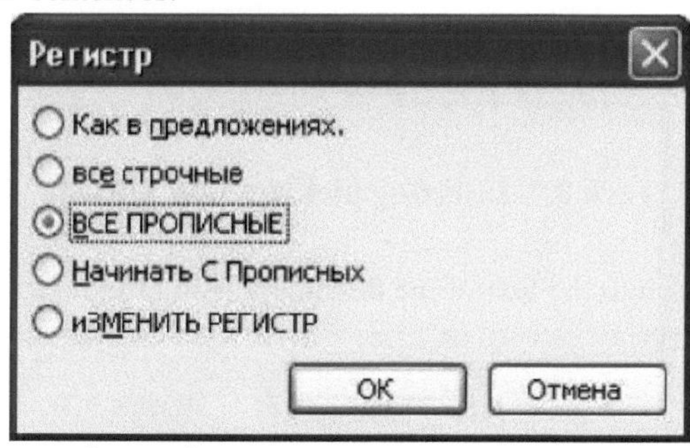

Figure 8.6. Text case formatting

Additional task

Task 8.6. Inserting WordArt objects into the text

Work order

1. Start the Microsoft Word text editor.
2. Use the *Insert/Drawing* command to run the programme WordArt (fig.8.7). In the *Edit* WordArt *Text* window, enter the title text (fig. 8.8).

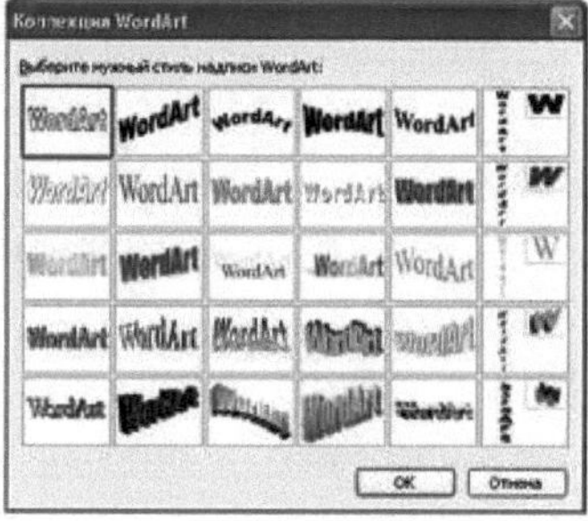

Fig.8.7. Inserting WordArt object into a document

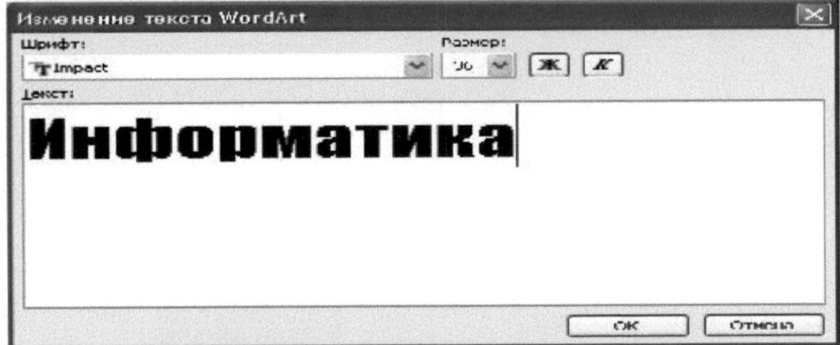

Fig.8.8. Text input window Use WordArt to create a title for the document:

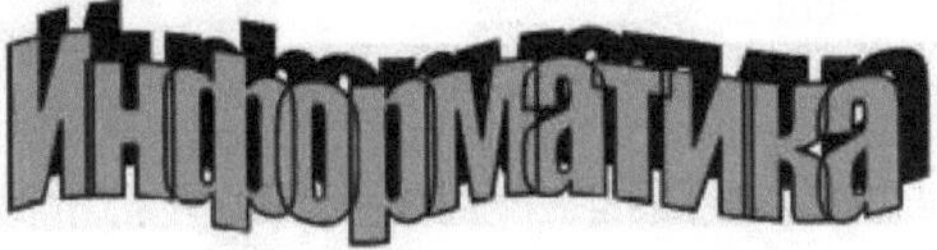

Task 8.7. Inserting pictures into the text

1. Insert 3 pictures into the text of the document using the Insert / Picture / Pictures commands:

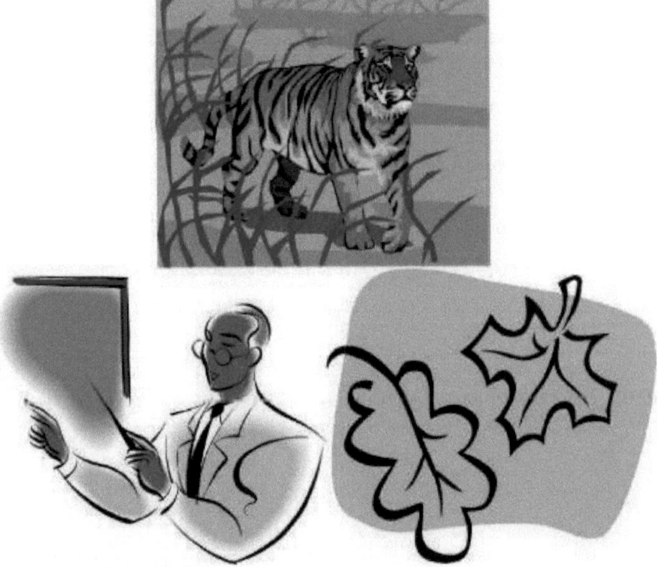

Task 8.8. Formatting figures

1. Open the "Document 3" file. Insert a drawing to study the formatting (Insert/Picture/Pictures). Set different types of text flow around the picture (select the picture with the *Format/Picture/Position* tab*)*. Notice how the position of the text changes in relation to the drawing.

2. Trim the drawing by 0.5 cm *(Format/Drawing/Drawing* tab*).*

3. Fill the background of the drawing *(Format/Drawing/'Colours* tab *and lines).*

4. Save the document in your folder with the name "Document 4" *(File/Save As).*

Task 8.9. Preparing a document for printing

Work order

1. Prepare the "Document 4" file for printing. Set page parameters (Fig. 8.9):

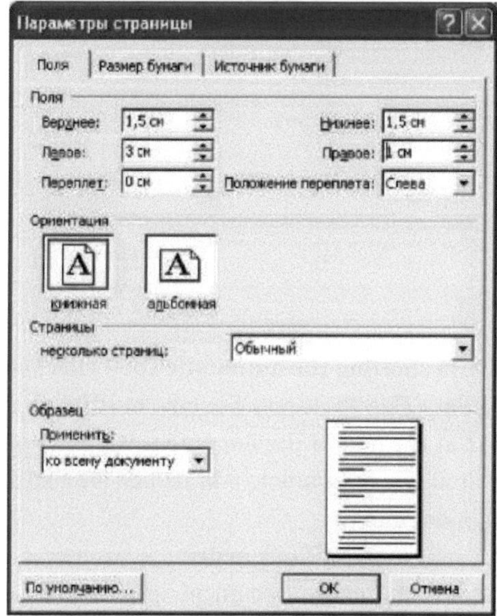

Fig. 8.9. Setting page parameters

2. Set page numbering *(Insert/Page Numbers),* position - top of page, alignment - right, with the number on the first page (Fig. 8.10).

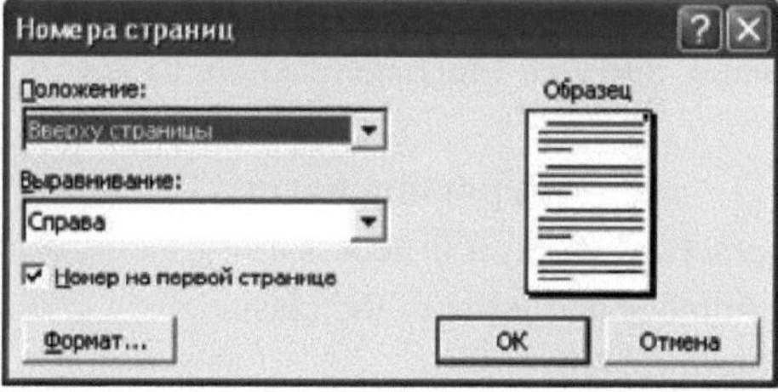

Fig.8.10. Setting page numbering 3. The spelling check is set by the *Service/Spelling* command or by the [F7] key.

5. **Set automatic spell checking *(Tools/Preferences/Spelling tab,* tick the**

"Automatically check spelling" checkbox (Fig. 8.11).

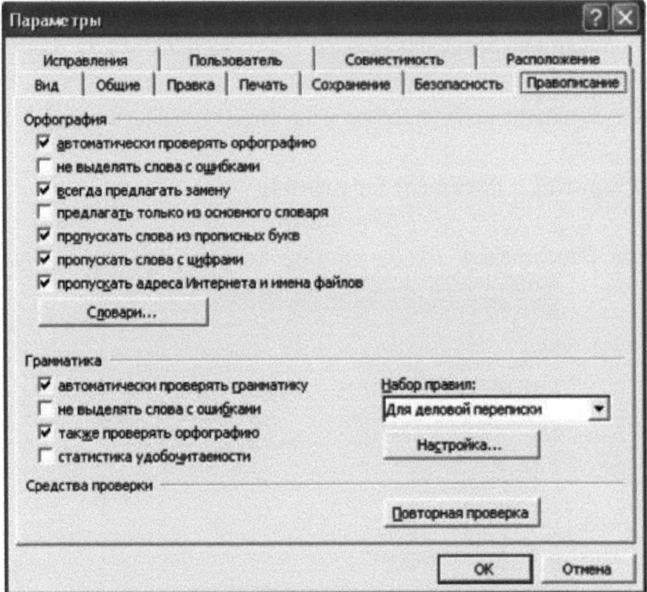

Fig. 8.11. Setting the automatic spell checker 5.

Preview the document (*File/Preview*). Specify multiple page previews. If a small portion of text at the end of the document is on a separate sheet,
Use the *Fit pages* button*, the* programme will reduce the font size and spacing.

Task 8.10. Printing a document

Work order

1. If you want to print the entire document in a single copy, use the *Print* toolbar button.
2. To print a range of pages or multiple copies, proceed as follows - File / Print. Set the page numbers to be printed to 1,3 and the number of copies to be printed to 2.
3. Print a fragment of the document. To do this, select the fragment, give the Format/Print command and set the page switch to the position - "Selected fragment".

Reporting Form:

When carrying out practical work, it is necessary to:

- Write down the number and topic of the class.
- Write down the assignment.
- Describe the performance of the work in detail.
- Answer the control questions.

Supervisory Questions:

1. What ways of creating lists do you know?
2. What is the best way to insert a letter into the text?
3. How to change the font case, text direction?
4. How do you break text into 3 columns?
5. How do I set the page parameters?

Recommended reading: 1.1,1.2, 2.2.

Practical work No. 9

ORGANISING CALCULATIONS IN MS EXCEL SPREADSHEET PROCESSOR.
FUNCTION UTILISATION

Purpose of the lesson. Study of information technology of organisation of calculations in MS Excel spreadsheets. Study of information technology of organisation of calculations using built-in functions in MS Excel spreadsheets.

Type of work: frontal

Lead time: 2 hours

Equipment: PC, Microsoft Excel

The chronological map of the lesson is 80 minutes.

Organisational part: cleanliness of premises, equipment, sanitary and hygienic conditions.

Student attendance is 2 minutes.

Assessment of students' knowledge : brief overview of the subject, questions and answers with students - 10 minutes.

Setting a new theme - 20 minutes.

Determination and consolidation of the level of mastery of the subject - 35 minutes.

Test questions - 10 minutes.

Homework - 3 minutes.

Practical work requirements:

1. answer the theoretical questions
2. organise the tasks in a practical workbook

Theoretical material

MS Excel is a universal system for performing calculations, searching and analysing data, for their graphical presentation.

An **MS Excel document** is a file with an arbitrary name and extension .xls, intended for data processing and storage. In MS Excel terms, such a file is called a workbook.

An **Excel workbook** is a set of worksheets saved in a single file. These can be worksheets, charts, slides, macros, dialogue sheets, or Visual Basic modules that allow you to use the Visual Basic language to develop macros for Excel. Worksheets refer to the main spreadsheet.

To perform tabular calculations, you need formulas. Since some formulas and their combinations are very common, Excel offers more than 200 preprogrammed formulas called functions.

All functions are categorised to make them easier to navigate. The built-in Function Builder helps you to use functions correctly at all stages of your work.

It allows you to create and calculate most functions in two steps.

The programme contains a complete alphabetically ordered list of all functions, in which you can easily find a function if you know its name; otherwise you should search by category. Many functions differ very slightly, so when searching by category, it is useful to use the short function descriptions offered by the Function Builder. A function operates on some data, which are called its arguments. A function argument can occupy a single cell or be placed in a whole group of cells. The function constructor provides assistance in defining any type of arguments. **Task 9.1. Create a table for calculating dollar exchange rate quotes**

The initial data are presented in Fig.9.1.

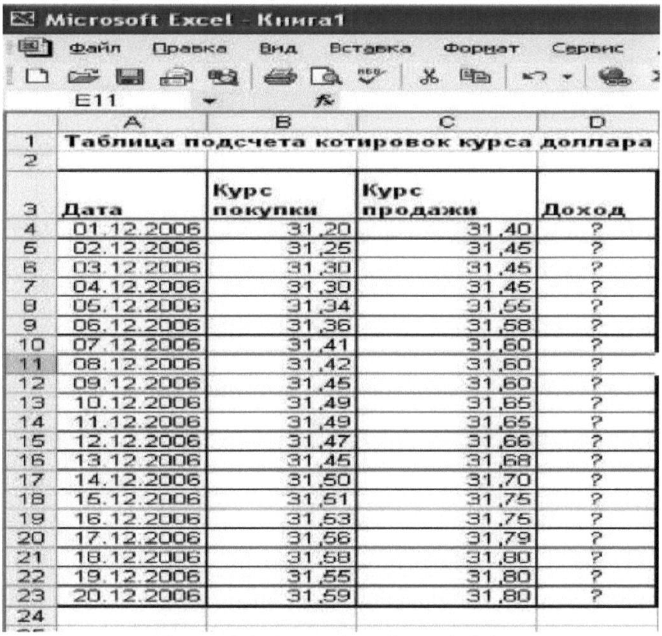

Microsoft Excel - Книга1

Файл Правка Вид Вставка Формат Сервис

E11

	A	B	C	D
1	**Таблица подсчета котировок курса доллара**			
2				
3	**Дата**	**Курс покупки**	**Курс продажи**	**Доход**
4	01.12.2006	31,20	31,40	?
5	02.12.2006	31,25	31,45	?
6	03.12.2006	31,30	31,45	?
7	04.12.2006	31,30	31,45	?
8	05.12.2006	31,34	31,55	?
9	06.12.2006	31,36	31,58	?
10	07.12.2006	31,41	31,60	?
11	08.12.2006	31,42	31,60	?
12	09.12.2006	31,45	31,60	?
13	10.12.2006	31,49	31,65	?
14	11.12.2006	31,49	31,65	?
15	12.12.2006	31,47	31,66	?
16	13.12.2006	31,45	31,68	?
17	14.12.2006	31,50	31,70	?
18	15.12.2006	31,51	31,75	?
19	16.12.2006	31,53	31,75	?
20	17.12.2006	31,56	31,79	?
21	18.12.2006	31,58	31,80	?
22	19.12.2006	31,55	31,80	?
23	20.12.2006	31,59	31,80	?
24				

Figure 9.1. Input data for task 9.1.

Work order

1. Launch the Microsoft Excel spreadsheet editor (on a standard MS Office installation, run *Start/Programs/Microsoft Excel)* and create a new eBook *(File/Create).* With a standard setup, the *Standard* and *Formatting* toolbars will open. If this does not happen, make a customisation *(Tools/Setup/Toolbars).*
2. Learn the purpose of Microsoft Excel toolbar buttons ("Standard" and "Formatting") by moving the cursor over them. Note that a number of buttons are similar to those in MS Word and perform the same functions *(Create, Open, Save, Print,* etc.).

3. Place the cursor on cell A1. Enter the title of the table "Dollar rate quote calculation table".

4. To design the table header, select the third row (by clicking on the row number), set word order by using the *Format/Cells/Cell Alignment tab/Replace by* words command, select horizontal and vertical alignment - "centre" (Fig. 9.2).

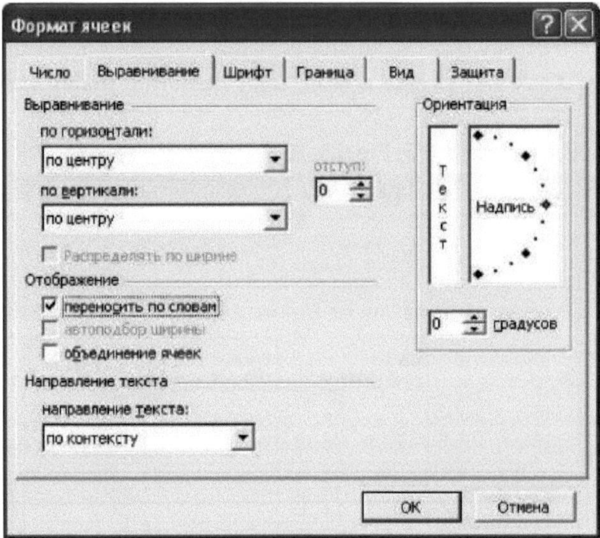

Figure 9.2. Setting word hyphenation when formatting cells

5. In the cells of the third row, starting from cell A3, enter the names of the table columns - "Date", "Buy rate", "Sell rate", "Income". Change the width of the columns from the main menu using the *Format/Column/Width* commands *while* moving the mouse in the row of column names (A, B, C, etc.).

6. Fill in the table with the initial data according to task 9.1.

To enter a range of date values, type the first date 01.12.06 and autocopy up to the date 20.12.06 (grab the autocomplete marker located in the lower right corner of the cell with the left mouse button and drag it down).

7. Format the values of the buy and sell rates. To do this, select the data block, starting from the upper left corner of the block (from cell B4) to the lower right corner (up to cell C23); open the *Format Cells* window using the *Format/Cell/Number tab* command and set the format to *Monetary,* currency designation - "no". Set the number of decimal places equal to 2 (Fig.9.3).

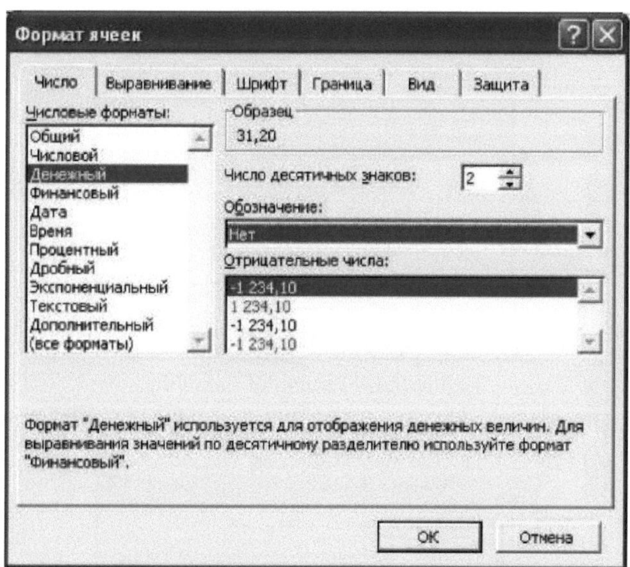

Fig. 9.3. Setting the format of numbers

Initially, a block of cells - the action object - is selected, and then a menu command is selected for execution.

To select a block of non-contiguous cells, you must first press and hold the [Ctrl] key while selecting the required areas.

8. Calculate in the column "Income" using the formula *Income = Selling rate - Buying rate,* in cell D4 type the formula = *C4-B4* (Latin letters are used in cell addresses). Enter the calculation formula in cell D4, then autocopy the formula.

To autocopy a formula, do the following: move the cursor to the autocomplete marker located in the lower right corner of the cell; when the cursor looks like a black cross, click the left mouse button and drag the formula down through the cells. You can autocopy by double-clicking on the autocomplete marker if there are no empty cells in the adjacent left column.

9. For cells with the result of calculations, set the format *Financial (Format/Cells/Number tab/Financial format,* currency sign - "p.", *number of decimal* places set to 2*).* - rubles, set the number of decimal places equal to 2).

10. Frame the table (Fig.9.4). To do this, select a block of table cells starting from the upper left or lower right corner of the table. Open the *Table Framing* window using *the Format/Cells/Borders tab* command. Set the maroon colour of the lines. Select a thin line for the inner lines and a thicker continuous line for the outline. The layout shows the final appearance of the border formatting, so click *OK* when you are satisfied with the appearance of the border in the layout.

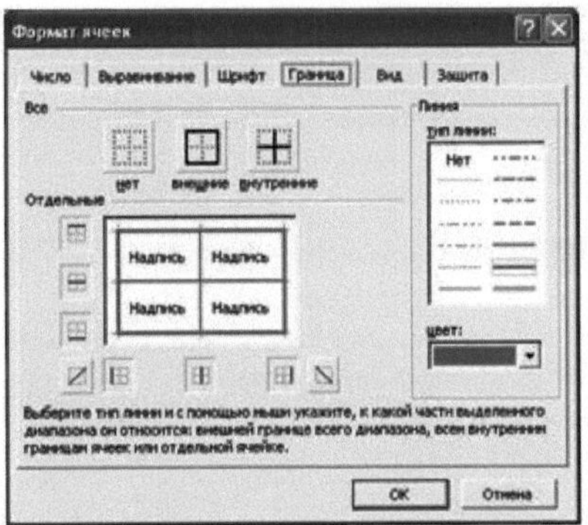

Figure 9.4. Framing of the table

11. Having selected the cells with the results of calculations, fill them with light blue colour *(Format/Cells/View tab) (Fig.9.*5).

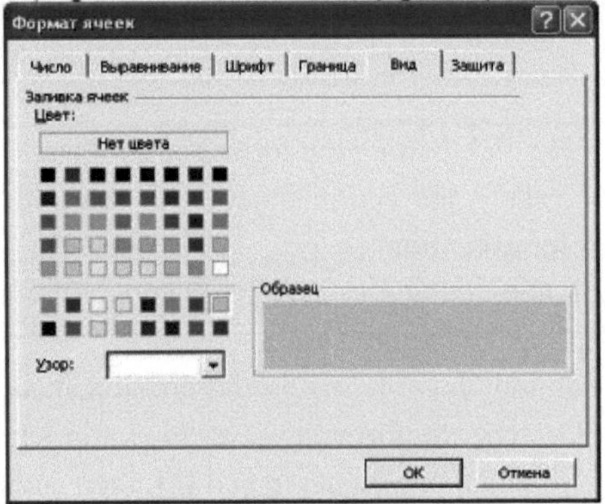

Figure 9. 5. Filling table cells

12. Format the table header. To do this, select the interval of cells from A1 to D1, merge them using the *Merge and centre* button of the toolbar or the menu command *(Format/Cells/ Alignment/Display tab - Merge Cells).* Set the font typeface to bold and the colour to your preference. The final view of the table is shown in Fig. 9.6.

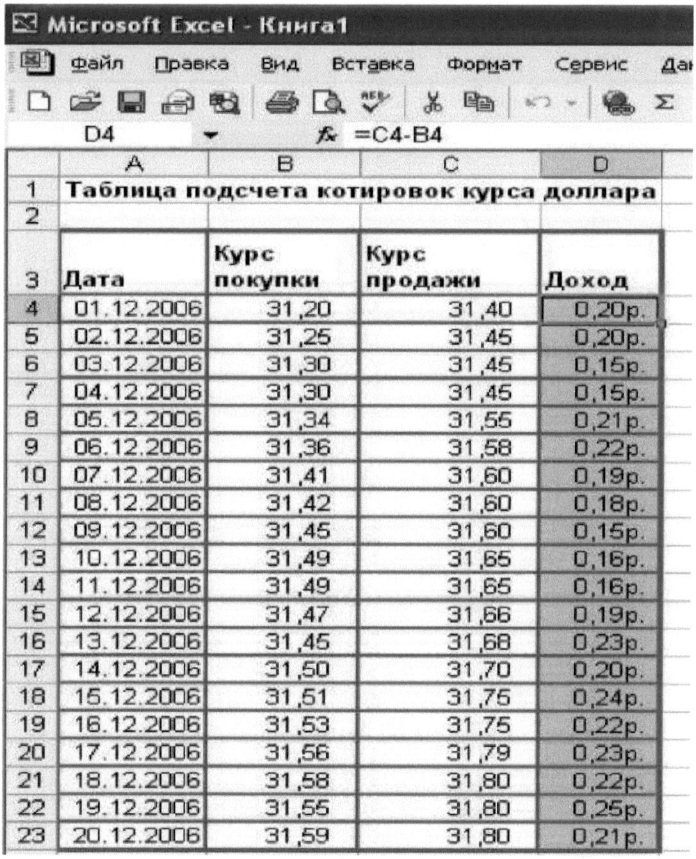

Microsoft Excel - Книга1

Файл Правка Вид Вставка Формат Сервис Да

D4 =C4-B4

	A	B	C	D
1	Таблица подсчета котировок курса доллара			
2				
3	Дата	Курс покупки	Курс продажи	Доход
4	01.12.2006	31,20	31,40	0,20р.
5	02.12.2006	31,25	31,45	0,20р.
6	03.12.2006	31,30	31,45	0,15р.
7	04.12.2006	31,30	31,45	0,15р.
8	05.12.2006	31,34	31,55	0,21р.
9	06.12.2006	31,36	31,58	0,22р.
10	07.12.2006	31,41	31,60	0,19р.
11	08.12.2006	31,42	31,60	0,18р.
12	09.12.2006	31,45	31,60	0,15р.
13	10.12.2006	31,49	31,65	0,16р.
14	11.12.2006	31,49	31,65	0,16р.
15	12.12.2006	31,47	31,66	0,19р.
16	13.12.2006	31,45	31,68	0,23р.
17	14.12.2006	31,50	31,70	0,20р.
18	15.12.2006	31,51	31,75	0,24р.
19	16.12.2006	31,53	31,75	0,22р.
20	17.12.2006	31,56	31,79	0,23р.
21	18.12.2006	31,58	31,80	0,22р.
22	19.12.2006	31,55	31,80	0,25р.
23	20.12.2006	31,59	31,80	0,21р.

Fig.9.6 Final view of the table

13. Rename the *Sheet* shortcut with the name "Dollar rate". To do this, double-click the shortcut and type a new name. You can use the *Rename* command of the shortcut's right-click context menu.

Task 9.2. Create a table for calculating the total revenue Order of work

The initial data are presented in Fig. 9.7

Microsoft Excel - Книга1

Файл Правка Вид Вставка Формат Сервис Данные Окно Справка OmniPage

Arial Cyr

E26

	A	B	C	D	E
1	Расчет суммарной выручки				
2					
3	Дата	Отделение 1	Отделение 2	Отделение 3	Всего за день
4	01 мая 2004 г.	1245,22	1345,26	1445,3	?
5	02 мая 2004 г.	4578,36	4326,97	4075,58	?
6	03 мая 2004 г.	2596,34	7308,68	6705,86	?
7	04 мая 2004 г.	1547,85	4628,74	7709,63	?
8	05 мая 2004 г.	3254,11	1948,8	6128,41	?
9	06 мая 2004 г.	1618,23	1245,85	4547,19	?
10	07 мая 2004 г.	3425,61	4685,21	2965,97	?
11	08 мая 2004 г.	921,02	8124,57	1384,75	?
12	09 мая 2004 г.	1057,85	11563,93	5928,24	?
13	10 мая 2004 г.	1617,33	4592,84	10471,73	?
14	11 мая 2004 г.	12457,5	7592,63	6459,99	?
15	12 мая 2004 г.	1718,02	4758,55	3784,12	?
16	13 мая 2004 г.	3462,85	6281,45	1108,25	?
17	14 мая 2004 г.	7295,84	3495,74	3475,25	?
18	15 мая 2004 г.	8285,2	710,03	6185,24	?
19	16 мая 2004 г.	6161,05	2845,22	9675,25	?
20	17 мая 2004 г.	9425,85	1675,85	13165,26	?
21	18 мая 2004 г.	9564,22	6425,85	3287,48	?
22	19 мая 2004 г.	2927,35	1237,25	4325,18	?
23	20 мая 2004 г.	6127,41	4352,88	2643,97	?
24	Итого:	?	?	?	?
25					
26					

Figure 9.7. Input data for task 9.2

1. Navigate to *Sheet2* by clicking on the *Sheet2* label,

This will open a new blank page of the eBook.

2. On *Sheet 2,* create a table for calculating total revenue according to the sample. In cell A4, set the date format as shown in Fig. 7 *(Format/Cells/Number tab/Numeric* format *Date,* select the date type with the month written as text - "1 May, 2004"). Next, copy the date down the autocopy column.

3. Type the words "Division 1" in cell BZ and copy them to the right into cells CZ and D3.

4. Highlight the area of cells B4:E24 and set the monetary format to two decimal places. Enter the numeric data.

5. Do the calculations in column "E".

Formula for calculation

Total for the day = Branch I + Branch 2 + Branch 3, in cell E4, type the formula = *B4 + C4 + D4.* Copy the formula to the entire column of the table. Remember that calculation formulas are entered only in the top cell of the column, and then they are

are copied down the column.

6. In cell B24, calculate the sum of column "B" data values (sum of column "Division 1"). To summarise a large amount of data, it is convenient to use the

Auto Summarise button *on the* toolbar. To do this, place the cursor in cell B24 and double-click on the Auto Sum button. The data of column "B" will be added.

7. Copy the formula from cell B24 to cells C24 and D24 by autocopying using the autocomplete marker.
8. Set lines around the table and format the created table and header.
9. Rename the *Sheet 2* label with the name "Revenue". To do this, double-click on the shortcut and type the new name. You can also use the *Rename* command of the shortcut's right-click context menu.
10. The result is an eBook with two tables on two sheets. Save the created e-book in your folder with the name "Calculations".

Task 9.3. Copy the table of dollar exchange rate quotations (task 16.1, sheet "Dollar exchange rate") and calculate the average, maximum and minimum values of dollar buying and selling rates under the table. Calculate the calculation using the "Function Wizard"

Work order

Copy the contents of the Dollar Rate sheet to a new sheet *(Edit/Move/Copy Sheet).* You can use the *Move/Copy* command from the shortcut context menu. Do not forget to tick the *Create* copy box for copying.

You can move and copy sheets by dragging their labels (hold down the [Ctrl] key to copy).

Quick Reference. To highlight the maximum/minimum values, place the cursor in the calculation cell, select Excel's built-in *MAX (MIN)* function from the Statistical category, highlight the range of column value cells B4: B23 as the first number (for the second calculation, highlight the range C4: C23).

Reporting Form:

When carrying out practical work, it is necessary to:

- Write down the number and topic of the class.
- Write down the assignment.
- Describe the performance of the work in detail.
- Answer the control questions.

Supervisory Questions:

1. Describe the functionality of the MS EXCEL spreadsheet processor.
2. What is an EXCEL book? What extension does the corresponding file have?
3. What is an EXCEL sheet?
4. How do I set print page options in EXCEL?
5. State the general rules for writing formulas in MS EXCEL.
6. Describe the algorithm for using the MS EXCEL function wizard.

Recommended reading: 1.1,1.2, 2.2.

Practical work No. 10

PLOTTING AND FORMATTING DIAGRAMS IN MS EXCEL

Class Objective. Study of information technology of data representation in the form of diagrams in MS Excel.

Type of work: frontal

Lead time: 2 hours

Equipment: PC, Microsoft Excel

The chronological map of the lesson is 80 minutes.

Organisational part: cleanliness of premises, equipment, sanitary and hygienic conditions.

Student attendance is 2 minutes.

Assessing student learning: a brief overview of the subject,
Q&A with students - 10 minutes.

Setting a new theme - 20 minutes.

Determination and consolidation of the level of mastery of the subject - 35 minutes.

Test questions - 10 minutes.

Homework - 3 minutes.

Practical work requirements:

1. Answer the theoretical questions
2. Organise the tasks in the practical workbook

Theoretical material

Diagram. Using the Diagram Wizard tool you can build diagrams of different types (graph, bar graph, pie chart). Depending on the selected type, the diagram may contain different elements. In most diagrams data is placed between two axes *OX* (arguments) and OU (values) and contains elements: axis captions (%, months), legends, diagram title, data markers, data rows, grid lines.

Task 1. Create a table "Calculation of the share of documented organisations" and build a pie chart based on the results of calculations

The initial data are shown in Fig. 10.1**, and the** results of the work are shown in Fig. 10.6.

Work order

1. Start the Microsoft Excel spreadsheet editor. Open the *Calculations* file created in Case Study 10 *(File / Open).*
2. Rename *the Sheet 3* label, giving it the name Specific Gravity.
3. On the "Specific weight" sheet, create the table "Calculation of the specific weight of documented organisations" using the sample as shown in Fig. 10.1.

Note. When entering text data starting with a dash or other mathematical sign, first press the *Space* key - text data sign, and then press the dash and text (state, -

municipal, etc.).

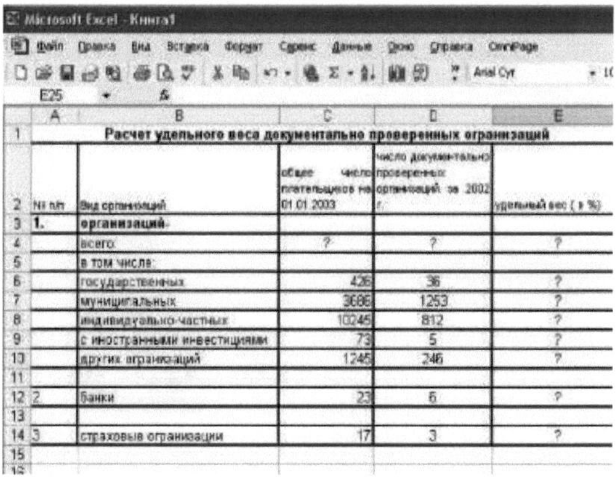

Расчет удельного веса документально проверенных организаций

№ п/п	Вид организаций	общее число плательщиков на 01.01.2003	число документально проверенных организаций за 2002 г.	удельный вес (в %)
1.	**организаций-**			
	всего:	?	?	?
	в том числе:			
	государственных	426	36	?
	муниципальных	3686	1253	?
	индивидуально-частных	10245	812	?
	с иностранными инвестициями	73	5	?
	других организаций	1245	246	?
2	банки	23	6	?
3	страховые организации	17	3	?

Fig. 10.1. Input data for task 10.3.

4. Do the calculations in the table. Formula for calculation
Specific weight = Number of audited organisations/Total number of payers.
In the Specific Weight column, set the percentage format of the numbers, and the software will multiply the data by 100 and add a percent sign.
5. Draw a diagram (pie chart) based on the results of the calculations using the diagram wizard.
To do this, select the interval of cells E7:E11 with the results calculation data and select the *Insert/Diagram* command.
At the first step of working with the diagram wizard, select the diagram type - *Pie chart (Volume version of the cut pie chart)* (Fig. 10.2).

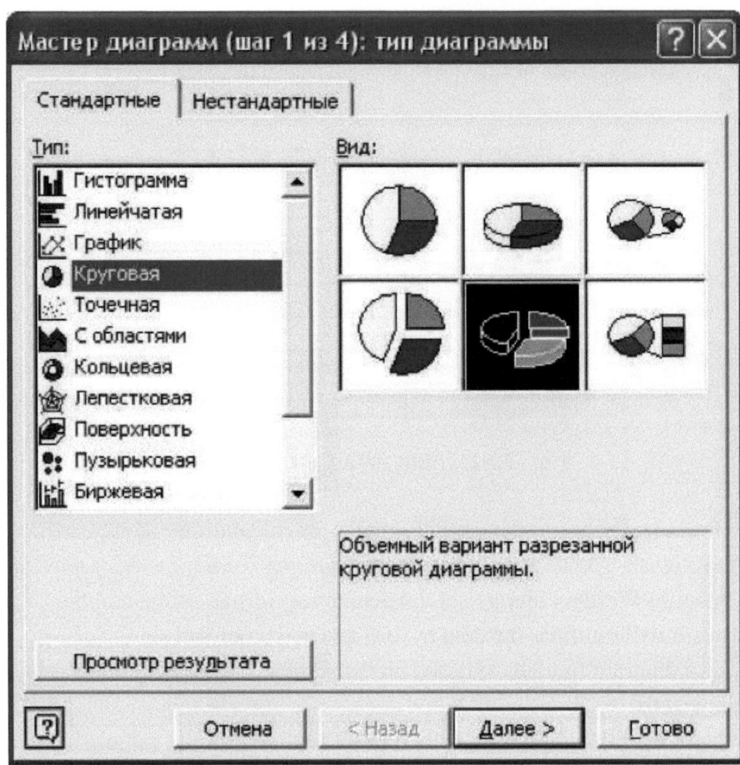

Fig. 10.2 Selecting the diagram type

In the second step, on the *Row* tab in the *Category captions* box, specify the interval of cells B7: B11 (Fig. 10.3).

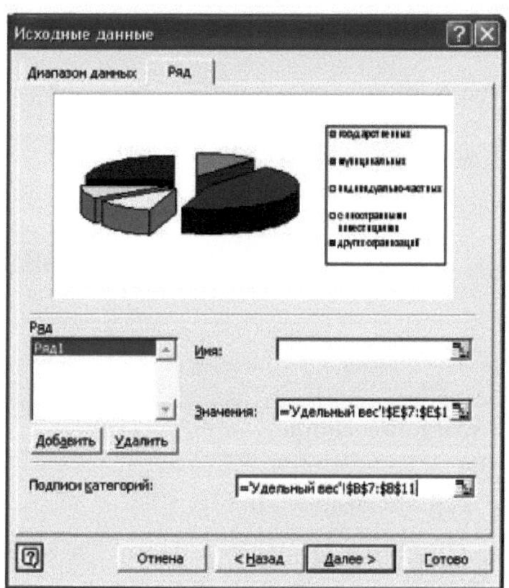

Fig. 10.3. Setting category captions when drawing diagrams

The third step of the diagram wizard. Enter the name of the diagram on the *Titles* tab; specify the value captions on the *Data captions* tab (Fig. 10.4).

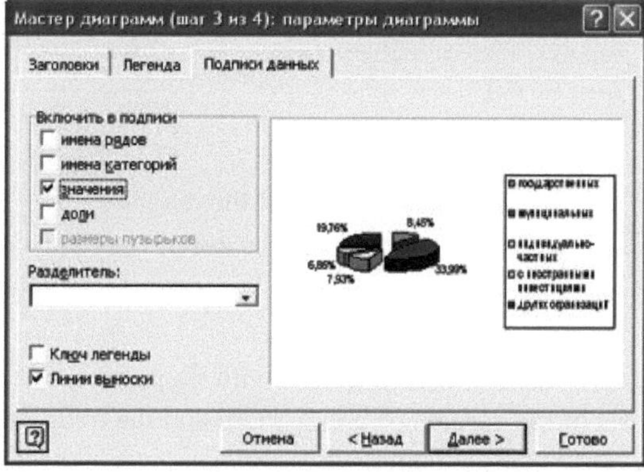

Fig. 10.4. Setting captions of pie chart values

The fourth step of the diagram wizard. Place the diagram on the existing sheet (Fig. 10.5).

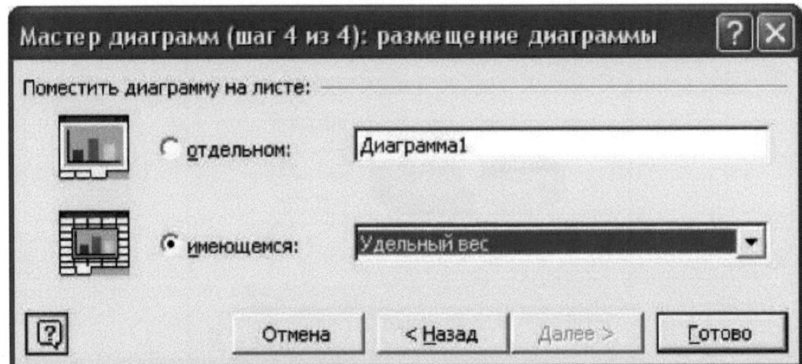

Fig. 10.5. Setting the diagram location

The final view of the diagram is shown in Fig. 10.6.

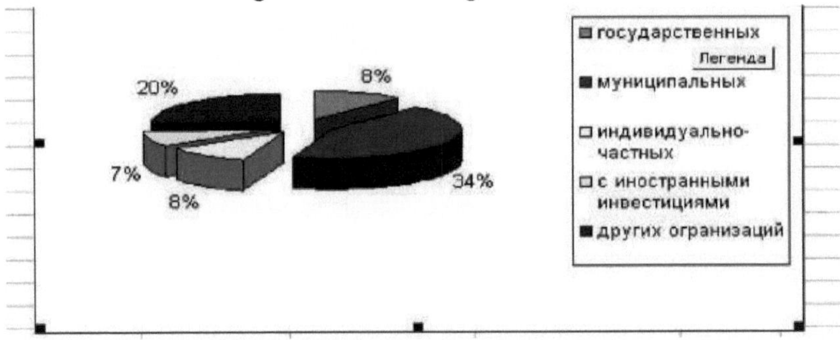

Fig. 10.6. Final view of the diagram

Task 10.2 Formatting the diagram "Calculation of the share of documented organisations"

Work order

1. Make the diagram active by clicking on it with the mouse, while doing so markers will appear at the corners of the diagram and the midpoints of the sides.
2. Move the diagram under the table with the mouse, resize the diagram (mouse over the markers).

Fill the background of the diagram. To do this, double-click on the diagram area. In the opened *Format* window of the *diagram area* (Fig. 10.7) select the yellow colour

and click the Fill *methods* button *(Fig.10.8).*

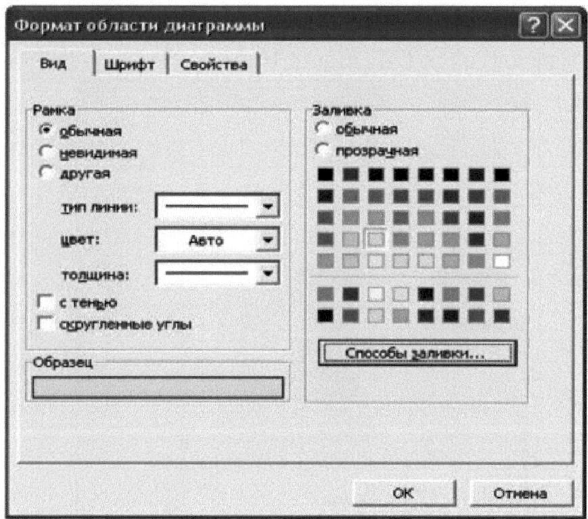

Fig. 10.7. Diagram area format dialogue window

3. In the *Fill Methods* window that opens, on the *Gradient* tab, use the slider to select the degree of shading and specify the hatch type *Vertical,* then click *OK* twice.

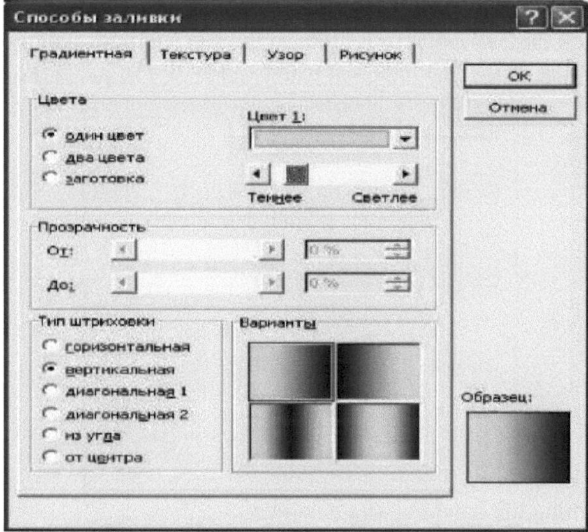

Fig.10.8. Fill methods dialogue window

4. Format the diagram legend (the box on the right side of the diagram). Click the mouse to make the legend area active, double-click to open the Legend *Format* window. On the *View* tab, click the *Fill Methods* button. In the *Fill*

Methods dialogue box that opens, select the *Texture* tab, specify the *White Marble* texture type and click *OK* (Figure 10.9).

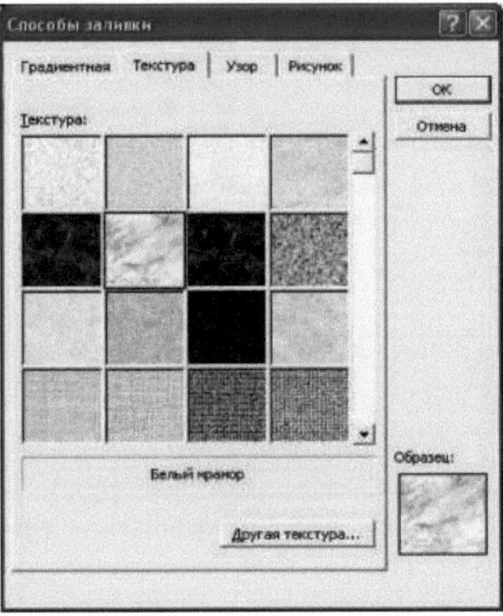

Fig. 10.9. Setting the legend background texture

5. Shade one sector (slice) of the pie chart. To do this, select one slice (perform two single clicks on the slice, the markers should move to the slice). Double-click on the selected slice to open the *Format data series* dialog box, select a colour and click the *Fill methods* button. In the *Fill* Methods window that opens, on the *Pattern* tab, select the diagonal hatch and click *OK* twice (Figure 10.10).

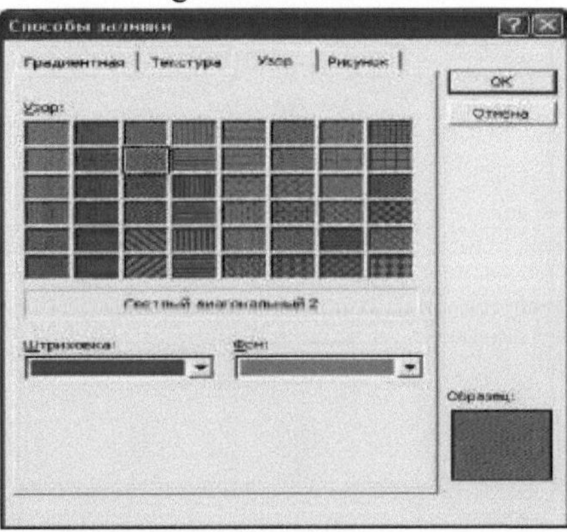

Fig. 10.10. Setting the hatching of a data item

6. Format the data captions (values 34%, 8%, etc.). To do this, double-click on one of the numeric values of data captions and in the opened window *Format of data captions* on the *Font* tab set: bold italics - 14 pt., font type - Anal Sug (Fig. 10.11).

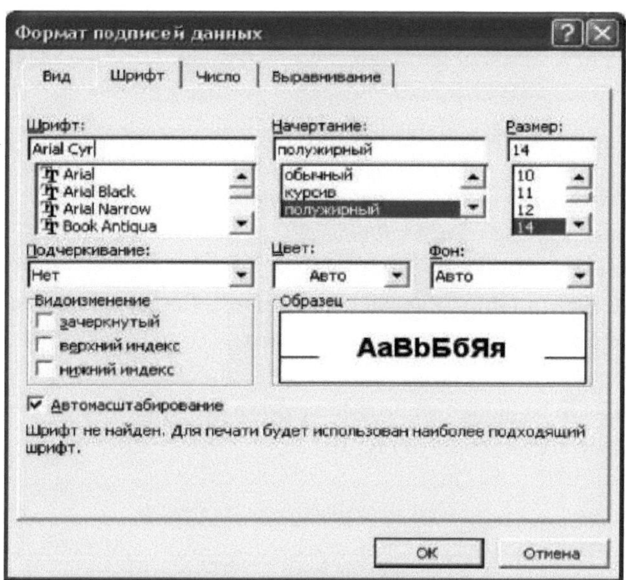

Figure 10. 11. Setting the format of diagram data captions

7. Enlarge the diagram area. To perform this formatting, click in the centre of the "layer cake" of the diagram, which will activate the diagram area. Change the size of the diagram construction area with the mouse by the corner markers.

8. Copy the created diagram (after selecting the diagram use the commands *Edit / Copy, Edit / Paste).*

9. Change the diagram type to a bar chart. To do this, make the diagram active by clicking the mouse, then right-click on the diagram area to call the Diagram *Properties,* select the *Diagram Type* command and specify the type - *Histogram.* Note the changes that have occurred in the diagram.

10. Perform the current file save *(File / Save).*

Task 10.3 Create a table "Summary of Plan Fulfilment". Build a graph and a diagram based on the results of calculations

Work order

The initial data are presented in Fig. 10.12.

Сводка о выполнении плана

Наименование	План выпуска	Фактически выпущено	% выполнения плана
Филиал №1	3465	3270	?
Филиал №2	4201	4507	?
Филиал №3	3490	2708	?
Филиал №4	1364	1480	?
Филиал №5	2795	3270	?
Филиал №6	5486	4587	?
Филиал №7	35187	2708	?
Филиал №8	2577	1480	?
Всего:	?	?	?

Fig. 10.12. Input data for task 10.3.

If necessary, new sheets of the ebook are added using *the Insert/Sheet* command.

Rename *the Sheet 4* label, giving it the name "Plan Execution".

Calculation formulas:

% of *plan fulfilment = Actual output/plan output;*

Total = sum of values for each column.

Perform the current file save *(File/Save).*

Task 10.4 Create a table "Payroll Calculation". Create a histogram and a pie chart based on the results of calculations

Work order

Select the data to be plotted while holding down the [Ctrl] key.

The initial data are presented in Fig. 10.13.

F19

	A	B	C	D	E	F
1		РАСЧЕТ ЗАРАБОТНОЙ ПЛАТЫ ЗА 1 КВАРТАЛ				
2						
3						ЗА ЯНВАРЬ
4	ФИО	Оклад	Премия 20%	Итого начислено	Подоходный налог 13%	Итого к выдаче
5	Баранова П.В.	15000	?	?	?	?
6	Васильев С.Н.	8000	?	?	?	?
7	Петрова А.Г.	11000	?	?	?	?
8	Петухова О.С.	9800	?	?	?	?
9	Савин И.Н.	12500	?	?	?	?
10						

Calculation formulas:

Bonus = Salary x *0.2;*

Total accrued = Salary + Bonus;

Income tax = Total accrued x *0.13;*

Total payable = Total accrued - Income tax.

Reporting Form:

When carrying out practical work, it is necessary to:

- Write down the number and topic of the class.
- Write down the assignment.
- Describe the performance of the work in detail.

- Answer the control questions.

Supervisory Questions:

1. Name the basic elements of an MS EXCEL processor diagram.
2. What types of diagrams can be created in MS EXCEL?
3. Describe the algorithm for creating a diagram in MS EXCEL.

Recommended reading: 1.1,1.2, 2.2.

Practical work No. 11

DESIGNING A DATABASE IN MS ACCESS SUBDATABASE

Class Objective. Studying the information technology of creating an empty database manually and with the help of templates using the wizard in the database management system (DBMS) Microsoft Access. Study of the objects of the training database "Borey".

Type of work: frontal

Lead time: 2 hours

Equipment: PC, Microsoft Access

The chronological map of the lesson is 80 minutes.

Organisational part: cleanliness of premises, equipment, sanitary and hygienic conditions.

Student attendance is 2 minutes.

Assessment of students' knowledge : brief overview of the subject, questions and answers with students - 10 minutes.

Setting a new theme - 20 minutes.

Determination and consolidation of the level of mastery of the subject - 35 minutes.

Test questions - 10 minutes.

Homework - 3 minutes.

Practical work requirements:

1. answer the theoretical questions
2. organise the tasks in the practical workbook

Theoretical material

MS Access is a component of MS Office designed to work with databases. When you start working with Access, a new database is created by assigning the original name and extension .mdb to the database file.

Each database has a database window. This window contains the *Objects* panel with the *Tables, Queries, Forms, Reports, Pages, Macros*, and *Modules* buttons. The database window also contains its own toolbar.

Basic Access database objects can be created in *Wizard* mode and in *Constructor* mode.

A **table** is used to store data in the form of records (rows) and fields (columns). Usually, each table is used to store the same type of data for a specific question.

Queries - allows you to set conditions for data selection and make changes to the data.

Forms - used for entering, viewing and editing information.

Pages *are* HTML files that allow you to view data using the Internet Explorer browser.

Reports - allow you to summarise and print information.
Macros - perform one or more operations automatically.
Modules - a programme to automate and configure database functions written in VB (Visual Basic) language.

Task 11.1 Creating an empty database

Work order

1. Start the Microsoft Access DBMS programme. To do this with a standard MS Office installation, run: *Start/Programs/ Microsoft Access*. In the *Microsoft Access* window that opens to open or select a database (DB), click *Cancel.*
2. Explore the programme interface by moving the mouse to different elements of the screen.
3. Select the *File/Create* command *.A* dialogue box will open on the screen *Creation* containing two tabs - *General* and *Databases* (Fig. 1.1):

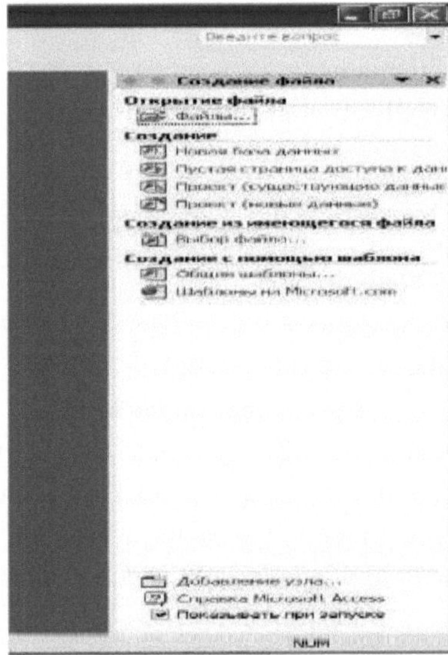

Fig. 11.1. Creation dialogue window

- The *General* tab is intended for creating a new empty database;
- The *Databases* tab allows you to create a database using the wizard and select a sample containing most of the database objects required for a certain subject.

4. Go to the *General* tab and click the *OK* button at the bottom of the dialogue box. *The New Database File* dialogue box will open on the screen (Fig. 11.2).
5. From the Folder drop-down list select the My Documents folder where you will save the database, and in the *File* name field enter the name of the database "My blank database" (you can enter your last name in the database name). The extension for the file name (mdb) can be omitted, because by default the *File*

Type input field is set to "Microsoft Access Database".

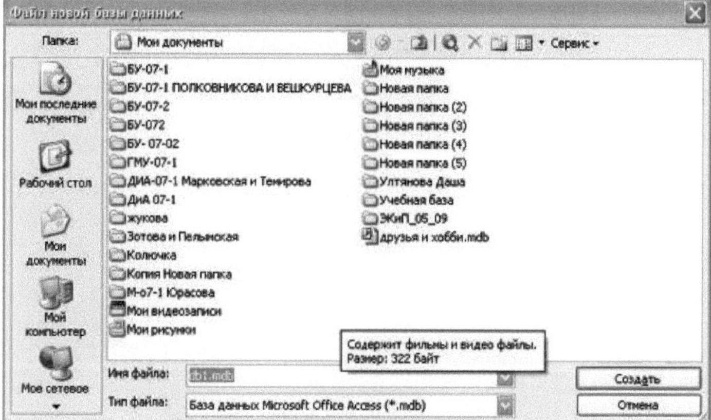

Fig. 11.2. New database file dialogue window

6. After entering the name of the database to be created, click the *Create* button. The *Database* window will open on the screen (Fig. 11.3). Study the interface of the database window.

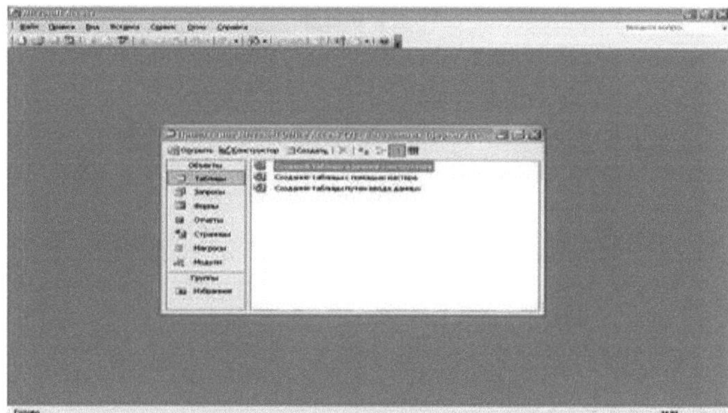

Fig. 11.3. New database window

7. Familiarise yourself with the properties of your database with the *Database Properties* command (Fig.11.4). Define the size of the created database.

Свойства: db1
Общие
Сводка
db1
Тип файла: Приложение Microsoft Access
Приложение: Microsoft Access
Изменить...
Размещение: C:\Documents and Settings\НАТАЛЬЯ\Мои докумен
Размер: 92,0 КБ (94 208 байт)
На диске: 92,0 КБ (94 208 байт)
Создан: 24 октября 2007 г., 19:13:02
Изменен: 24 октября 2007 г., 19:13:05
Открыт: 24 октября 2007 г., 19:13:05
Атрибуты: Только чтение Скрытый
Другие...
OK
Отмена
Применить

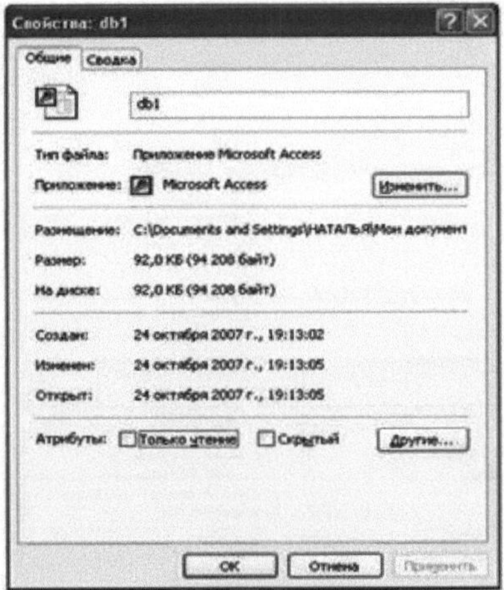

Fig. 11.4. Database property window

8. Close the empty database you created.

Task 11.2. Creating an empty database using templates using the wizard tools

Work order

1. Select the *File/Create* command or press the [Ctrl]-[N] keys. *The Create* dialogue box containing two tabs will open on the screen.

2.. Click the Create with template - Common templates tab.

The list of databases (templates) offered by the wizard will appear on the screen (Fig. 11.5).

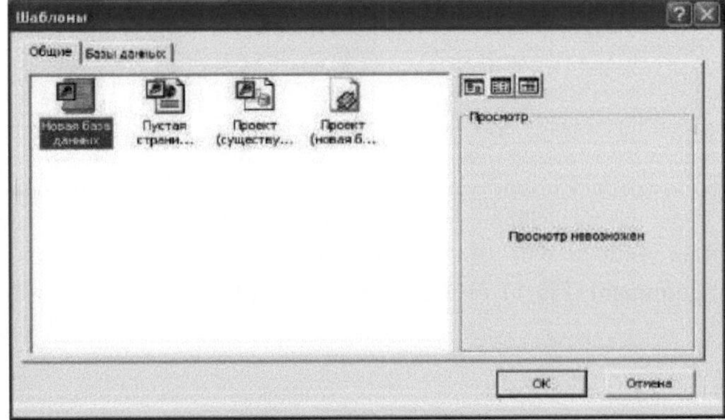

Fig.11.5. *Database* tab

3. Select the "Contacts" sample database from the list and start the database wizard by pressing the *OK* button.

4. In the Folder drop-down list, select the My Documents folder

where you want to save the database, enter the name of the My Contacts database in the *File* name field, and then click *Create.*

5. In the next dialogue window the wizard tells what information the database to be created will contain (Fig. 11.6).

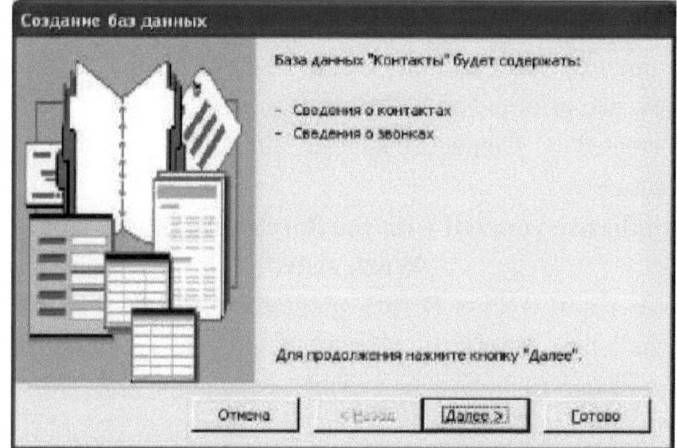

Fig.11.6. Dialogue window with information about the created base

The following buttons are located at the bottom of the window:

Cancel - terminates the wizard;

Back - allows you to return to the previous step in the wizard;

Next - allows you to proceed to the next step in the wizard's work;

Done **-** starts the wizard to create the base with the set parameters.

Click the *Next* button to continue.

6. The opened dialogue window (Fig. 11.7) contains two lists. The first one is the list of database tables, the second one is the list of fields of the selected table. Usually the fields that will be included in the table are marked in the list, but you can include additional fields by marking them in the list. To go to the next window of the wizard, click *Next.*

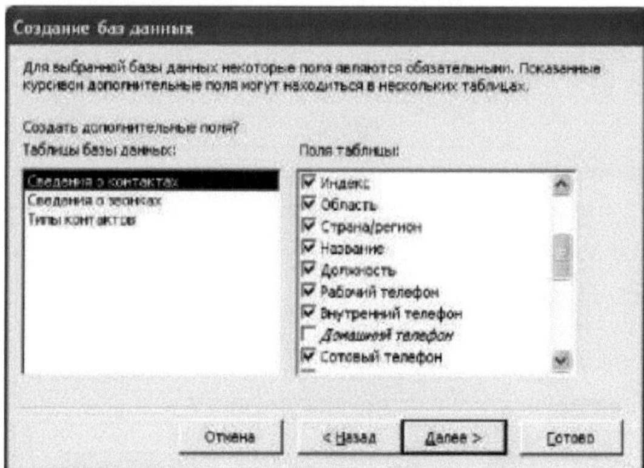

Fig. 11.7. Selection from the list of database table fields

7. In the following windows, select the screen layout, the type of reports you want to create, the title, and the figure that will appear on all reports.

8. After clicking *Finish* in the last window, the wizard proceeds to creating a database consisting of tables with the fields you have specified, forms for entering and viewing information, and reports. After the database creation process is completed, you can immediately use the ready database: enter data into tables, view and print them.

9. Close the created Contacts database and DBMS Microsoft Access.

Task 11.3 Familiarise yourself with the Boreas training database

Work order

1. Start the Microsoft Access DBMS programme. To do this with a standard MS Office installation: *Start/Programs/Microsoft Access. Open the Borey.mdb file from the database window, which is located on the C:\Program Files\Microsoft Office\OFFICE11\SAMPLES disc.*

2. After opening the Boreas database , a window will appear on the screen with a brief characteristic of the base (Fig.11.8). Press the *OK* button.

Вашему вниманию предлагается учебная база данных "Борей", созданная для изучения Microsoft Access. Поработайте с ее данными и используйте ее формы, отчеты и другие объекты в своих собственных приложениях.
Все объекты базы данных доступны из окна базы данных. Для добавления описаний объектов в окне базы данных выполните команду "Таблица" из меню "Вид".
БОРЕЙ
ТОРГОВАЯ КОМПАНИЯ
Больше не выводить заставку
OK
Названия компаний, товаров и персонажей, а также приведенные данные являются вымышленными и не представляют любое реальное лицо, товар или организацию, если не оговорено иное.

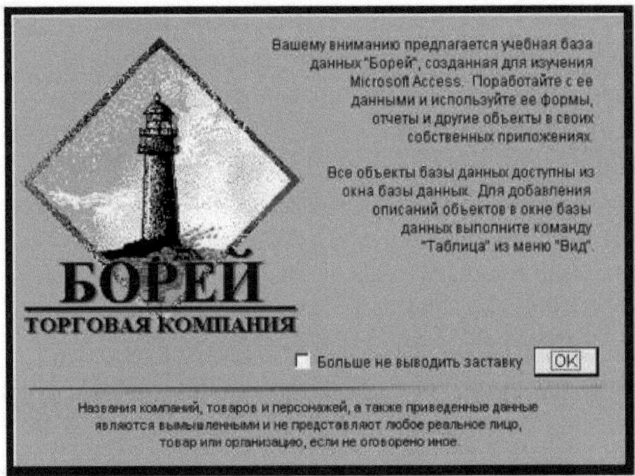

Fig. 11.8. Database Characterisation window

3. Set the tabular view of the screen *(View/Table)* to display a brief description of the base objects (Fig. 11.9).

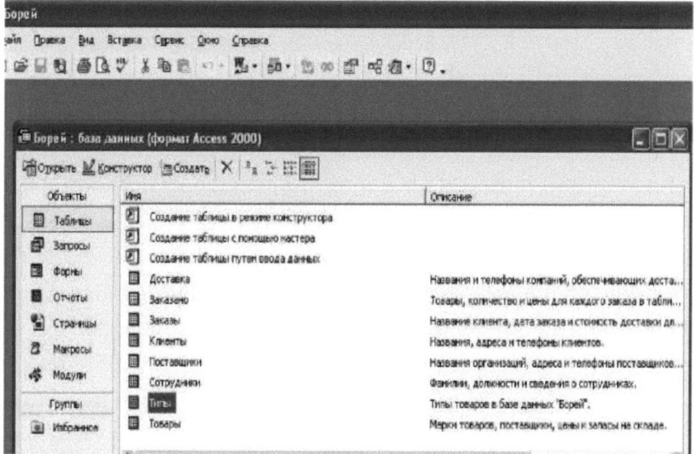

Fig. 11.9. Borey base table with description

4. Examine the structure of the Boreas database by switching the tabs of the database objects - *Tables, Queries, Forms, Reports.* On the *Tables* tab, calculate the number of tables in the "Boreas" database. Study the links between the tables. To do this, call the data schema *using the Service/Data Schema* command or the *Data Schema* button (Fig. 11.10).

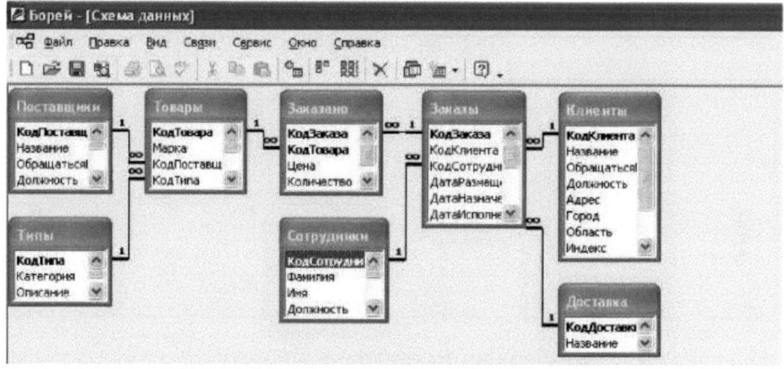

Fig. 11.10. Data schema of the Borey base

Identify which tables the Goods table is linked to.

5. Select the base object - *Tables.* Open the "Orders" table by double-clicking the mouse or using the *Open* button. Determine the number of records and fields in it. The number of records is displayed at the bottom of the table window to the right of the record control buttons.

6. Sort by customers in the "Orders" table. To sort, place the cursor in the *Customer* field and execute *the Records/Sorting/Sort in ascending* order command. Count the number of orders of the first customer in the list.

7. Filter the data of the table "Orders" by the date of order placement located in

the upper record (row). To filter, select the date in the top row of the table and execute *the Records/Filter/Filter by Selection* command. Notice how the table view has changed - you can see data related to only one date. Remove the filter *{Records/Remove Filter).* Close the Orders table.

8. Open the table "Clients". Determine the total number of clients (at the bottom of the "Clients" table window to the right of the record control buttons) (Figure 11.11). The figure shows that there are 91 clients.

9. Find London in the *City* field. To do this, place the cursor in the *City* field and execute *the Edit/Find* command. In the *Search and Replace* window that opens (Figure 11.12), on the *Search* tab, enter the word "London" as a sample and click *Find Next.* The search will be performed and the cursor will be positioned on the name of the city - London. Close the Find and Replace window.

Клиенты : таблица

Код клиента	Название	Обращаться к	Должность	Адрес	
ALFKI	Alfreds Futterkiste	Maria Anders	Представитель	Obere Str. 57	Бе
ANATR	Ana Trujillo Emparedados	Ana Trujillo	Совладелец	Avda. de la Constitucion 2222	Мє
ANTON	Antonio Moreno Taqueria	Antonio Moreno	Совладелец	Mataderos 2312	Мє
AROUT	Around the Horn	Thomas Hardy	Представитель	120 Hanover Sq.	Ло
BERGS	Berglunds snabbkop	Christina Berglund	Координатор	Berguvsvagen 8	Лу
BLAUS	Blauer See Delikatessen	Hanna Moos	Представитель	Forsterstr. 57	Ма
BLONP	Blondel pere et fils	Frederique Citeaux	Главный менеджер	24, place Kleber	Ст
BOLID	Bolido Comidas preparadas	Martin Sommer	Совладелец	C/ Araquil, 67	Ма
BONAP	Bon app'	Laurence Lebihan	Совладелец	12, rue des Bouchers	Ма
BOTTM	Bottom-Dollar Markets	Elizabeth Lincoln	Бухгалтер	23 Tsawassen Blvd.	Тс
BSBEV	B's Beverages	Victoria Ashworth	Представитель	Fauntleroy Circus	Ло
CACTU	Cactus Comidas para llevar	Patricio Simpson	Продавец	Cerrito 333	Бу
CENTC	Centro comercial Moctezuma	Francisco Chang	Главный менеджер	Sierras de Granada 9993	Мє
CHOPS	Chop-suey Chinese	Yang Wang	Совладелец	Hauptstr. 29	Бе
COMMI	Comercio Mineiro	Pedro Afonso	Ученик продавца	Av. dos Lusiadas, 23	Са
CONSH	Consolidated Holdings	Elizabeth Brown	Представитель	Berkeley Gardens	Ло
DRACD	Drachenblut Delikatessen	Sven Ottlieb	Координатор	Walserweg 21	Ах
DUMON	Du monde entier	Janine Labrune	Совладелец	67, rue des Cinquante Otages	На
EASTC	Eastern Connection	Ann Devon	Продавец	35 King George	Ло
ERNSH	Ernst Handel	Roland Mendel	Менеджер по продажам	Kirchgasse 6	Гр
FAMIA	Familia Arquibaldo	Aria Cruz	Помощник менеджера	Rua Oros, 92	Са
FISSA	FISSA Fabrica Inter. Salchichas S.A.	Diego Roel	Бухгалтер	C/ Moralzarzal, 86	Ма
FOLIG	Folies gourmandes	Martine Rance	Помощник продавца	184, chaussee de Tournai	Ли
FOLKO	Folk och fa HB	Maria Larsson	Совладелец	Akergatan 24	Бр
FRANK	Frankenversand	Peter Franken	Главный менеджер	Berliner Platz 43	Мі
FRANR	France restauration	Carine Schmitt	Главный менеджер	54, rue Royale	На
FRANS	Franchi S.p.A.	Paolo Accorti	Представитель	Via Monte Bianco 34	Ту
FURIB	Furia Bacalhau e Frutos do Mar	Lino Rodriguez	Менеджер по продажам	Jardim das rosas n. 32	Ли
GALED	Galeria del gastronomo	Eduardo Saavedra	Главный менеджер	Rambla de Cataluna, 23	Ба

Запись: 1 из 91

Уникальный пятисимвольный код, образуемый из названия организации. NUM

Fig. 11.11. Table "Clients" of the "Borcy" base

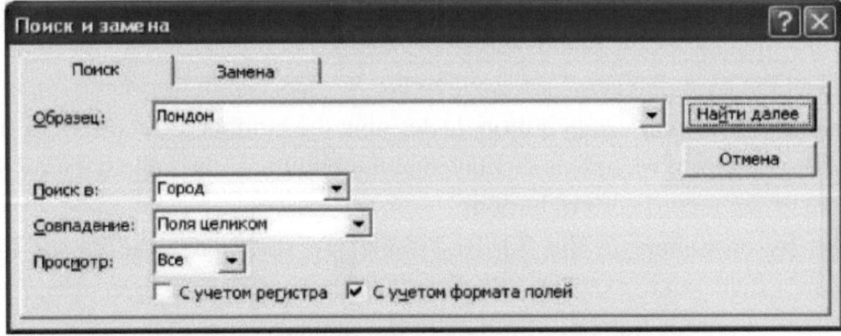

Fig. 11.12. Search by pattern in a table field

10. Filter for clients from London (in the *City* field, highlight the word "London" and follow the commands *Records/Filter/Filter by Selection).* Count the number of clients from London. Remove the filter *(Records/ Remove Filter).* Sort by client name (descending).

11. Open the table "Goods" in the *Builder,* to do this, place the cursor on the table "Goods" and click the *Builder* button (Fig. 11.13).

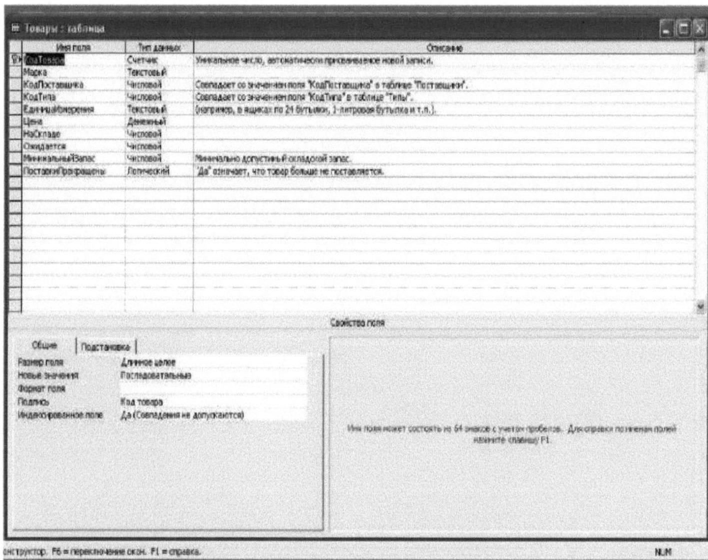

Fig. 11.13. Window Constructor of the table "Goods"

Take a close look at the appearance of *the Table Builder.* In the upper part of the table there is a table with the name of fields, their data type and description. Determine which field is the key field. The lower part displays the field properties.

12. Close the "Borey" database and MS Access DBMS.

Additional task

Task 11.4. Create the "Orders" database using a template using the wizard tools

Examine the relationships between the database tables *(Service/Data Schema). Enter any 10 records into the Orders table.*

Reporting Form:

When carrying out practical work, it is necessary to :

- Write down the number and topic of the class.
- Write down the assignment.
- Describe the performance of the work in detail.

- Answer the control questions.

Supervisory Questions:

1. Formulate the definition of "Database Management System".
2. List the types of basic Access database objects and their purpose.
3. What is a key field, what is its purpose?
4. What is the purpose of inter-table links and what are their types?

Recommended reading: 1.1,1.2, 2.2.

Practical work No. 12

CREATING TABLES AND CUSTOM FORMS FOR DATA ENTRY IN MS ACCESS SUBDAS

Class Objective. Studying the information technology of creating tables and user forms for data entry in DBMS Access.

Type of work: frontal

Lead time: 2 hours

Equipment: PC, Microsoft Access

The chronological map of the lesson is 80 minutes.

Organisational part: cleanliness of premises, equipment, sanitary and hygienic conditions.

Student attendance is 2 minutes.

Assessment of student knowledge: brief overview of the course, questions and answers with students - 10 minutes.

Setting a new theme - 20 minutes.

Determination and consolidation of the level of mastery of the subject - 35 minutes.

Test questions - 10 minutes.

Homework - 3 minutes.

Practical work requirements:

1. answer the theoretical questions
2. organise the tasks in the practical workbook

Theoretical material

Tables are the main objects of any database, which store all the data available in the database, as well as the structure of the database (fields, their types and properties). All other objects (forms, reports, queries) depend on these tables.

Creation of tables using the wizard is performed by selecting a standard table ("Employees", "Orders", etc.) and required fields from a standard table or several standard tables. The selected field names can be edited. After entering the table name, a key field is selected, which allows you to make connections between tables in the database.

When creating a table in the *Constructor* mode, an empty table structure is displayed, in which you should enter the names of indicators, specify the data types in the fields and set the field sizes. In the lower part of the table structure form, you can set the table field properties that allow you to change the ways of storing and displaying data.

Database table fields do not just define the structure of the database - they also define group properties of the data written to the cells belonging to each field.

The main properties of database table fields are listed below, using Microsoft Access as an example.

Task 12.1 Create the "Students" table using the table creation wizard. Use the "Students" table as a template

Work order

1. Start the Microsoft Access DBMS programme and open the new database "My Empty Database".

2. In the database window, select "Tables" as the object. Create a table with the help of the wizard . To do this, select command *Create table using the wizard* (Fig. 12.1) or click the *Create/Table Wizard/OK* button.

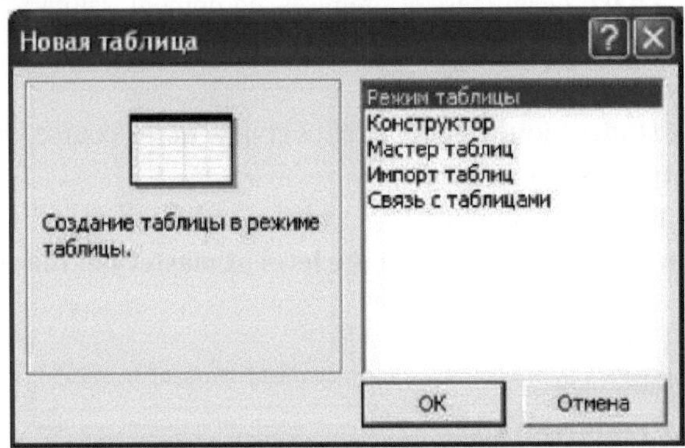

Fig.12.1. Selecting the table wizard when creating a new table

3. In the *Create Tables* dialogue box that opens (Fig. 12.2), select "Students" as the table sample. From the sample fields, select the fields (use the arrow buttons of the *Select One/All Fields* dialogue box*)* in the specified sequence:

First name, Middle name, Last name, Position, Address, Telephone number, Specialisation.

Click the *Next* button.

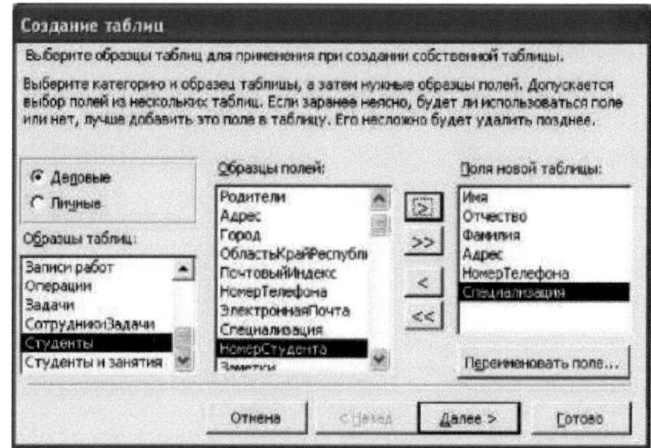

Fig. 12.2. Selection of fields from the sample table "Students"

4. Set the table name to "Students". Set the switch to "Automatic hatch detection in Microsoft Access". Click *Next.* In the next *Wizard* window, in the "Next steps after creating the table" select *Enter data directly into the table. Done.*
5. The wizard will automatically create a key field, and a new field *Student Code* with the data type "Counter" will be created. Open the "Students" table in the *Constructor* and make sure that a key icon appears to the left of the "Code" field name - the key field mark.
6. Switch to the table mode *(View/Table mode).* Move the *Last name* field to the left of the *First name* field. To move a field, select it by clicking on its name and drag the field to the new location by its name.
7. Enter eight records (rows) in the "Students" table according to the sample (Fig. 12.3).

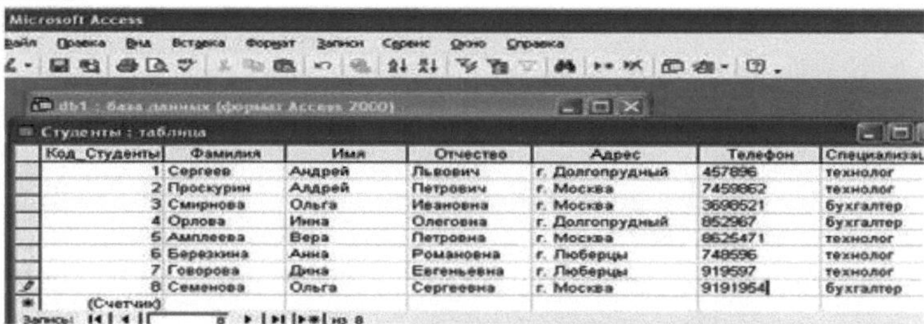

Код_Студенты	Фамилия	Имя	Отчество	Адрес	Телефон	Специализац
1	Сергеев	Андрей	Львович	г. Долгопрудный	457896	технолог
2	Проскурин	Андрей	Петрович	г. Москва	7459862	технолог
3	Смирнова	Ольга	Ивановна	г. Москва	3698521	бухгалтер
4	Орлова	Инна	Олеговна	г. Долгопрудный	852967	бухгалтер
5	Амплеева	Вера	Петровна	г. Москва	8625471	технолог
6	Березкина	Анна	Романовна	г. Люберцы	748596	технолог
7	Говорова	Дина	Евгеньевна	г. Люберцы	919597	технолог
8	Семенова	Ольга	Сергеевна	г. Москва	9191954	бухгалтер
(Счетчик)						

Fig. 12.3. Table "Students" 8. Save the table.

Task 12.2: In the same database, create a table "Students and assignments" in table mode

Work order

1. Select the *Create table by entering data* command or click the *Create/Table Mode* button - Fig. 12.4.

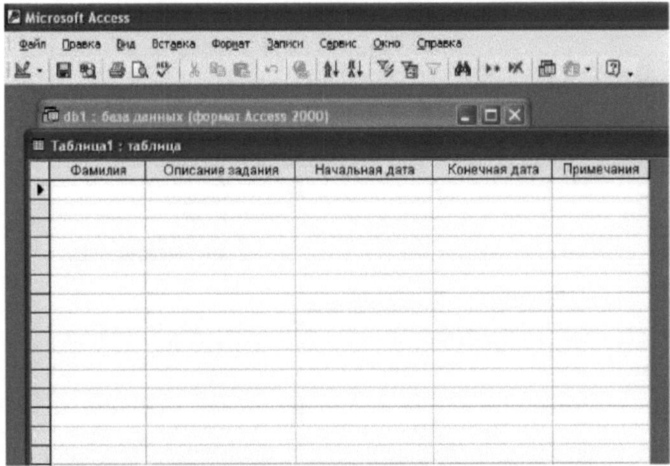

Fig. 12.4. View of the table created in the Table mode

2. Rename the fields in the table by assigning them names: *Last Name, Job Description. Start date, End date, Notes.*

Quick Reference. To change the field name, double-click on the field name and enter a new name.

3. Save the table with the name "Students and Assignments".

4. When saving, the programme will ask you if you want to create a key field? Click *Yes* to create a key field and a new field *Code* with data type *Code* will be created

"Counter". Open the table in the *Builder* and make sure that a key icon appears to the left of the field name "Code" - a key field mark.

5. Copy students' surnames from the "Students" table to the "Students and assignments" table. To copy, go to the "Students" table, select the *Surname* field and execute the *Edit/Copy* command.

surnames will be written to the memory buffer. After that, open the "Students and assignments" table, select the *Surname* field and execute *the Edit./Paste* command. Make sure that the surnames appear in the field of the "Students and tasks" table.

6. Go to the *Constructor* mode (Fig. 12.5). Set the data type for the *Start date* and *End date* fields - "Date/Time", field format - *Short date format*.

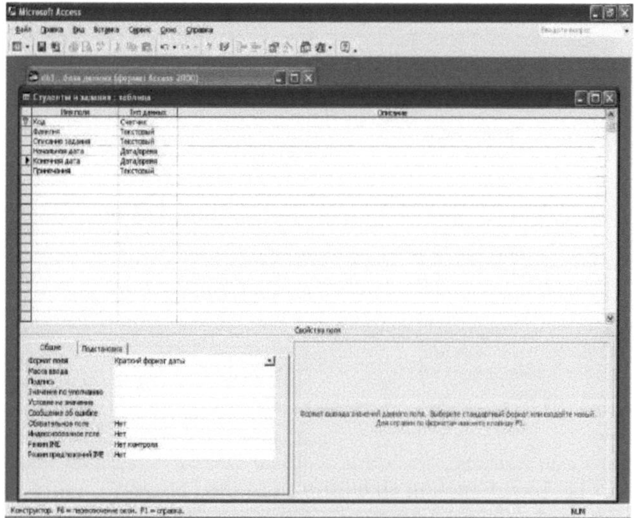

Fig. 12.5. Setting the data type - Date/Time

7. Enter the data in the "Students and assignments" table using the template provided

in Figure 12.6.

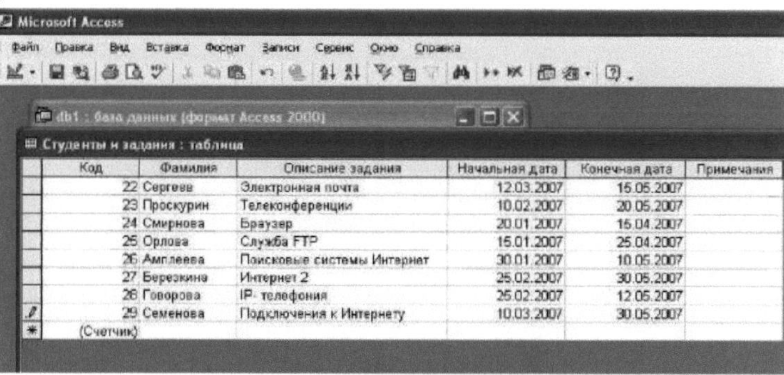

Fig. 12.6. Final view of the table "Students and tasks"

8. Perform the current save of the "Students and classes" table and close the table.

Task 12.3 Create an autoform in the same database to a column on the "Students" table. *A form* is a database object that displays data from tables or queries. A form is intended mainly for data entry.

Work order

1. Select the base object - *Forms*. Click the *Create* button, in the *New Form* window that opens, select the form type: "Autoform: per column"; specify the "Students" table as the data source (Fig. 12.7). Save the created form with the

name - "Students".

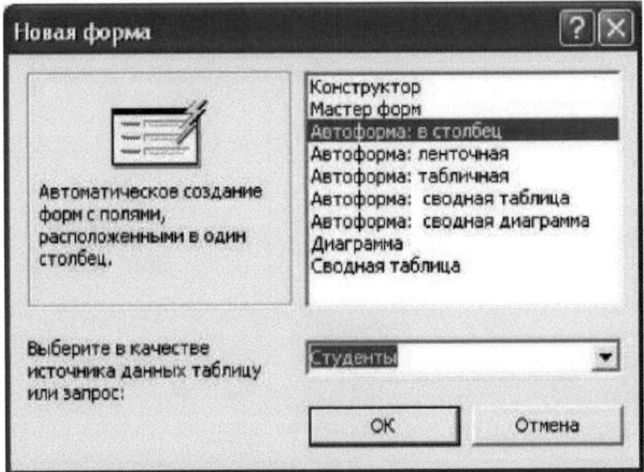

Fig. 12.7. Creating an autoform of the "Students" table

2. Using the record buttons at the bottom of the window, navigate to the last record, then to the first record.

3. Enter two new records using the "Students" form (Fig. 12.8). To enter a new record, use the record operation buttons at the bottom of the window.

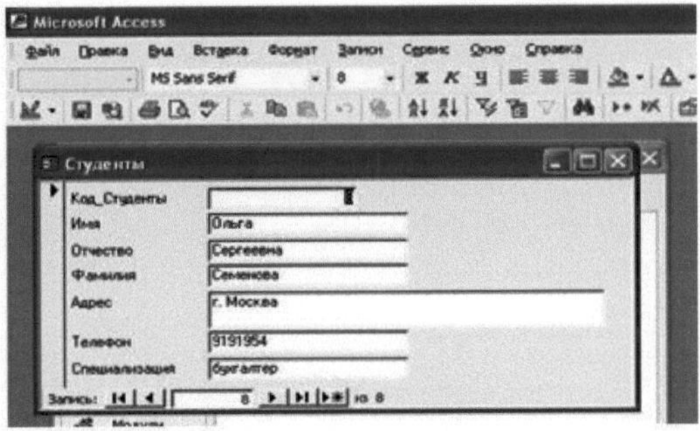

Fig. 12.8. Autoform "Students"

4. Save the created form with the name "Students".

Task 12.4 Create a form in the same database using the form wizard based on the "Students and Assignments" table

Work order

1. To create a form using the wizard, select the base object - *Forms.* Click the *Create* button; in the *New Form* window that opens, select the form type - Forms Wizard; specify the Students and Assignments table as the data source.

2. Select the fields -First name*, Job description, End date* (Fig. 12.9)

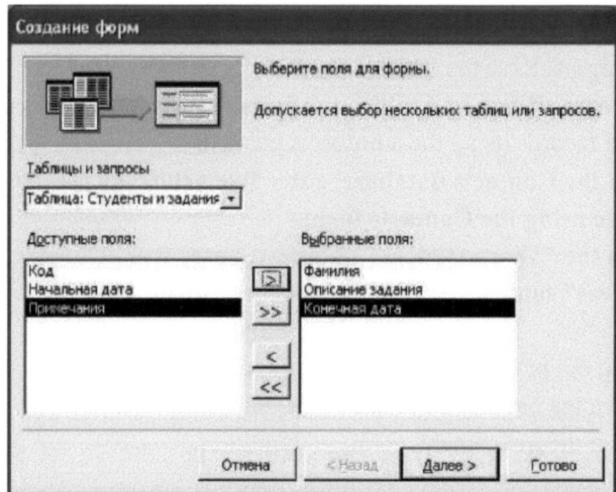

Fig. 12.9. Selecting fields when creating a form using the form wizard

Use the *Select One/All* Fields buttons between the selection windows to select fields;

form appearance - in one column;

the style is formal;

the name of the form is Students and Assignments.

3. In the form mode *(View/Form* Mode*)* add several records. Use the buttons at the bottom of the window to navigate through the records and create a new record.

4. Save the created form with the name "Students and Assignments".

5. Use the Form Wizard to create the "Students and Assignments 1" form based on all fields of the "Students and Assignments" table. Compare the appearance of the created form with the "Students and Assignments" form. Enter three new records using the Students and Assignments form.

Additional tasks

Task 12.5: In the same database, create a table "Session Results" using the table creation wizard with the following fields: "Surname", "Group", "Economics", "Philosophy", "Mathematics", "Notes".

Work order

1. Select fields independently from different samples, applying the possibility of renaming fields.
2. Perform automatic creation of a key field when saving the table. In the *Constructor* mode check the type of created fields.
3. Copy the students' last names from the Students table.

Enter five records in the table mode into the created table "Session Results". Preview the Session Summary table in Preview mode and place it on a single sheet. You will probably have to set the sheet to landscape orientation and reduce the margins. Save the table.

Task 12.6 Create ribbon and table autoforms for the table "Session Totals"

Enter multiple records using the autoforms created.

Task 12.7: In the Contacts database, enter five arbitrary records in the Contacts table using the Contacts form

Task 12.8: In the "Work Orders" database, enter five arbitrary records in the "Employees" table using the "Employees" form

Reporting Form:

When carrying out practical work, it is necessary to:

- Write down the number and topic of the class.
- Write down the assignment.
- Describe the performance of the work in detail.
- Answer the control questions.

Supervisory Questions:

1. Give the definition of a table.
2. List and briefly characterise the main modes of table creation.
3. What ways of creating shapes do you know?
4. What is a form mode?

Recommended reading: 1.1,1.2, 2.2.

Practical work No. 13

MODIFYING TABLES AND WORKING WITH DATA USING QUERIES IN MS ACCESS SUBDATA

Class Objective. Studying the information technology of modifying database tables and creating queries and reports in DBMS Access.

Type of work: frontal

Lead time: 2 hours

Equipment: PC, Microsoft Access

The chronological map of the lesson is 80 minutes.

Organisational part: cleanliness of premises, equipment, sanitary and hygienic conditions.

Student attendance is 2 minutes.

Assessing student learning: a brief overview of the subject,
Q&A with students - 10 minutes.

Setting a new theme - 20 minutes.

Determination and consolidation of the level of mastery of the subject - 35 minutes.

Test questions - 10 minutes.

Homework - 3 minutes.

Practical work requirements:

1. Answer the theoretical questions
2. Organise the tasks in the practical workbook

Theoretical material

Queries are objects that are used to extract data from tables and provide them to the user in a convenient form. Queries are used to perform such operations as data selection, sorting and filtering, as well as data transformation according to a specified algorithm, creation of new tables, automatic filling of tables with data imported from other sources, performing calculations and many others. Different types of queries are created for different actions.

A select query is designed to select data stored in tables and does not modify that data.

A change query is used to modify or move data. This type includes: a query to add records, a query to delete records, a query to create a table, and a query to update.

A query with a parameter allows you to define one or more selection conditions at query runtime.

A number of queries are built using wizards. The following types of queries can be created:

a simple query that allows you to select fields from multiple tables or queries;
cross-query calculates sum, mean, number of elements and values of other statistical functions, grouping data and outputting them in a compact form;
repeated records search for identical records in any field in the table;
records without subordinates find all records that do not have corresponding records in another (linked) table.

Task 13.1 Modification of the "Students" table

Work order

1. Launch the Microsoft Access DBMS programme and open the database you created in the previous lesson.
2. Open the "Students" table and edit it: - in the second or third record (depending on your gender), change the last name to your own;
- copy the entry with the last name "Orlova" to the ninth;
- enter a new record in the *Data Entry* mode *{Records/Data Entry).* Note that data filtering has taken place and all records are invisible; - return the table to its normal appearance; to do this, remove the filter (*Records/Delete Filter)*;

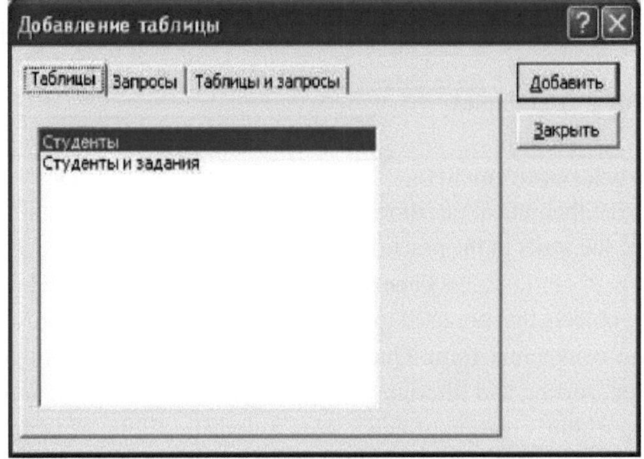

- select all students with the name "Andrei" (by filtering on the highlighted one);
- select all students from the city of "Lyubertsy";
- select all students of the specialisation "Technologist".

3. Add new fields to the Students table before the *Specialisation* field: *Scholarship, Overhead.* To do this, make the *Specialisation* field current or select it and use the *Insert/Column* command. Assign appropriate names to the created fields - "Scholarship" and "Overhead".

{ "overhead".

4. Go to the *Constructor* mode *(View/Constructor)* and check and, if necessary,

change the data types of the created fields (the created fields must have numeric or monetary data type). Return to the Table mode *(View/Table mode).*

5. Fill in the *Scholarship* field with numerical data in the amount of P450.
6. Close the Students table.

Task 13.2 Calculate the values of the "Overhead" field in the "Students" table by creating an update request. The allowance is 35% of the scholarship

Work order

1. To fill in the *Overhead* field, select the object - *Queries,* call the query form with the command *New/Constructor.*Quick Reference. A query form is a form designed to define a query or filter in *Constructor* mode or in the *Advanced Filter* window. In previous versions of Access, the term "pattern-based query form" (QBE) was used. In the opened dialogue window *Add Table*, select the table "Students", click the *Add* button and close this window (Fig. 13.1), and the *List of fields of* the table "Students" will be added to the query form (Fig. 13.2). By default, the selection query form will open.

Fig. 13.1. Adding the list of fields of the "Students" table

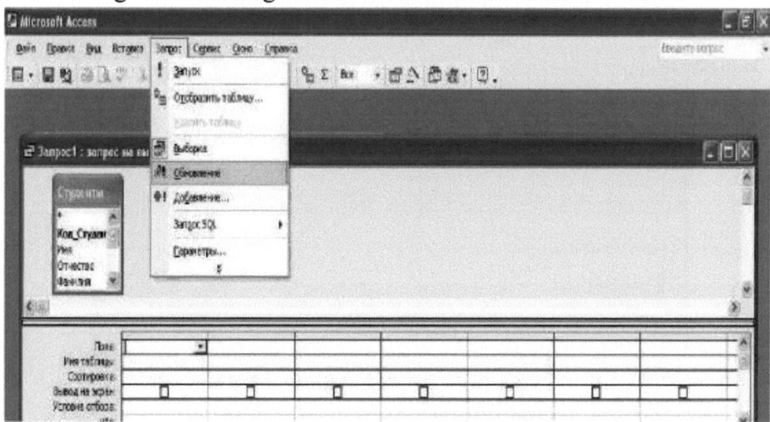

Figure 13. 2. Sample request form

Quick Reference. *Field List* (in form and report) - a small window containing a list of all fields in the underlying record source. In Microsoft Access database, it is possible to display the list of fields in the *Form, Report and Query Builder* mode, as well as in the *Data Schemes* window.

2. From the *Query* menu, select the *Update* command. Notice the changes in the request type form *(Sorting* has changed to *Update).*

From the list of fields in the query form, drag the field to be updated - *Overhead;* in the "Update" line, enter the calculation formula to fill in the

Overhead field (Fig. 13.3).

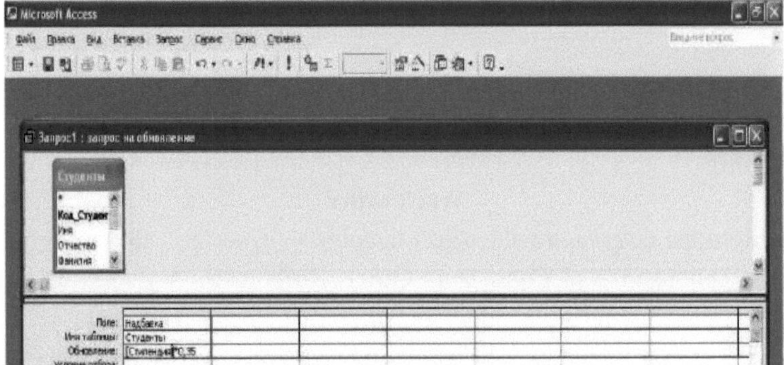

Fig.13.3. Query form for calculating the Overhead field

Since the Overhead is 35% of the Stipend, type in the Update line to calculate *the Overhead* field:

[Scholarship] * 0.35.

Quick reference. Field names are enclosed in square brackets when typing a formula in the "Update" line.

4. Perform the *Update on request by* launching the request for execution using the *Request/Run* command or the *Run* button in the toolbar (in the form of an exclamation mark). Confirm the execution of the request with the *Yes* button in the dialogue box that opens.

5. Save the request under the name "Overhead" (Fig. 13.4).

Fig.13.4. Setting the name of the request when saving

6. Open the "Students" table and check if the calculations are correct. If everything is done correctly, the *Overhead* field will be filled with the values of 157,50 p.

7. Change the sequence of fields: place the *Specialisation* field before *Scholarship.* The moving rules are the same as in all Windows applications (select the *Note* field*,* drag it to a new location with the mouse).

8. Save the changes in the table. If necessary, create a backup copy of the database on a floppy disc.

Task 13.3: Search for repeating records by the "Name" field of the

"Students" table

Work order

1. Select the database object - *Queries*. Click the *Create* button, in the *New Query* window that opens, select the type of query - "Recurring records" (Fig. 13.5).

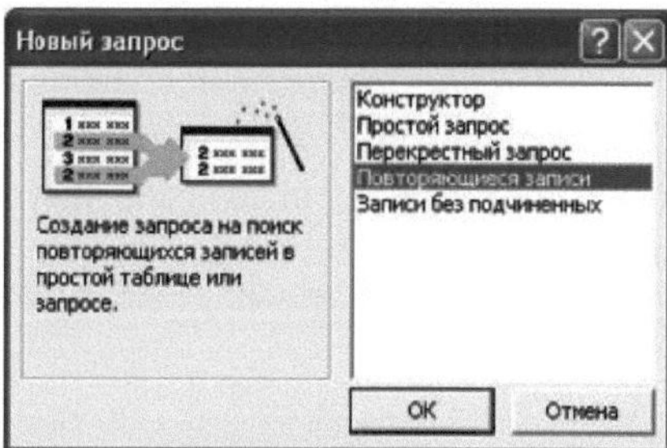

Fig. 13.5. Creating a query to search for repeated records

2. Specify the "Students" table as the data source (Fig. 13.6).

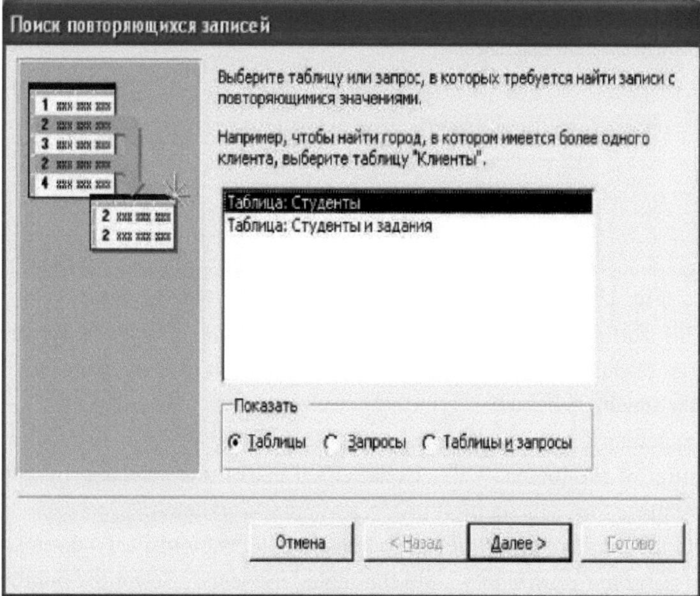

Fig. 13.6. Selecting the "Students" table as a source of repeating records

3. In the following dialogue boxes, select the field by which the repeated records will be searched - *Name,* select the *Surname* and *Specialisation* fields as additional fields. As a result, the records of repeating students' names will be selected, and information about students' surnames and specialisation will be added to them. Save the query under the name "Repeating records".

Task 13.4. Requests for selection by condition

Work order

1. Select from the table "Students" the surnames, first names and telephone numbers of all students whose surname begins with the letter "C".

To do this, select the base object - *Queries.* In the *Constructor* mode create a query for selection *{Create/Constructor).* Add the table "Students".

2. Select the *Surname, First Name, Phone Number* fields from the list of table fields. In the "Selection condition" line of the *Surname* field of the query form type the condition - "C*" (the * symbol indicates the presence of arbitrary characters after the letter "C") (Fig. 13.7).

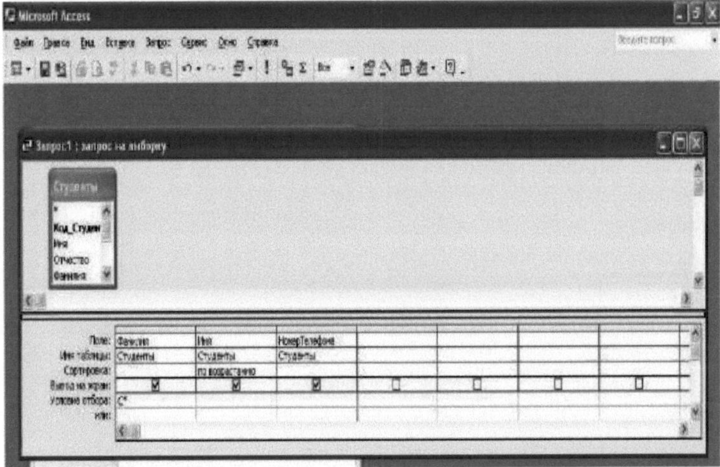

Fig. 13.7. Selection of surnames beginning with the letter "C"

3. Set the sorting by the *Name* field. Check that the "Output to screen" line, which is responsible for outputting the records in the dynamic set to the computer screen, is ticked.

After launching the query for execution using the *Query/Run* command or the *Run* button of the toolbar ("!" - exclamation mark), the selection by condition will take place. Save the request under the name "Surname C".

4. Select all employees with the specialisation "technologist". To do this, create a query *(Create/Constructor).* Add the table "Students". Select the output fields *Surname, First Name, Middle Name, Specialisation.* In the "Selection Condition" line of the *Specialisation* field of the query form, type the condition - "technologist". Set sorting in ascending order for the *Surname* field.

To run the request, select the *Request/Run* command. Save the request under the name "Request - Technologist" (Fig. 13.8).

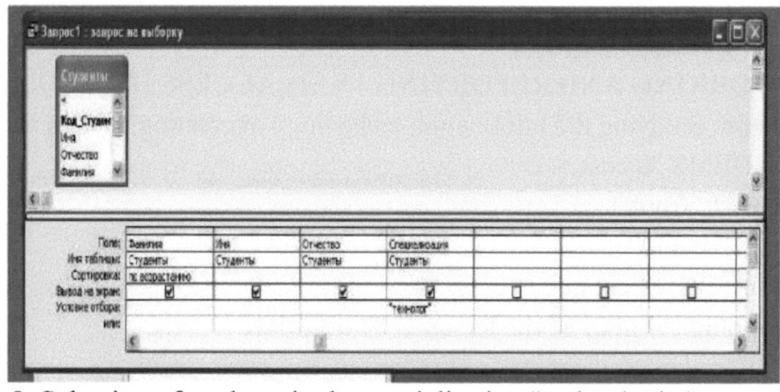

Fig. 13.8. Selection of students in the specialisation "technologist"

Additional tasks

Task 13.5: In the same database, create a query to select from the "Students and Assignments" table all students who received assignments later than 20.02.07 (in the field "Students and Assignments"). "Start date" set the selection condition > 20.02.07)

Task 13.6: In the same database, create a query on the "Students and Assignments" table to search for repeated records by the "End date" field

Reporting Form:

When carrying out practical work, it is necessary to:

- Write down the number and topic of the class.
- Write down the assignment.
- Describe the performance of the work in detail.
- Answer the control questions.

Supervisory Questions:

1. List and characterise the main types of Access database queries.
2. What is the purpose of a query-selection?
3. Where is query-change used?
4. What allows you to define a query with a parameter?
5. What queries can be built using the wizard?

Recommended reading: 1.1,1.2, 2.2.

Practical work No. 14

DATA WORKING AND REPORTING IN MS ACCESS DBMS Objective of the lesson. Studying the information technology of creating queries and reports in DBMS Access.

Type of work: frontal

Lead time: 2 hours

Equipment: PC, Microsoft Access

The chronological map of the lesson is 80 minutes.

Organisational part: cleanliness of premises, equipment, sanitary and hygienic conditions.

Student attendance is 2 minutes.

Assessment of student knowledge: brief overview of the course, questions and answers with students - 10 minutes.

Setting a new theme - 20 minutes.

Determination and consolidation of the level of mastery of the subject - 35 minutes.

Test questions - 10 minutes.

Homework - 3 minutes.

Practical work requirements:

1. Answer the theoretical questions
2. Organise the tasks in the practical workbook

Theoretical material

Reports. In terms of their properties and structure, reports are similar to forms in many respects, but they are intended only for outputting data, not on the screen, but on a printing device (printer). In this regard, reports differ in that they have special measures for grouping the output data and for displaying special design elements typical for printed documents (header and footer, page numbers, service information about the time of report creation). Reports can contain data from several tables or queries.

You can create reports of the following types:

- a simple printout from *Table* or *Form* mode, used as a draft report;
- detailed report - a well-prepared report in a visual user-friendly form, including a number of additional elements;

- A special report that allows for the preparation of, for example, postal mailings.

stickers and letter forms.

Task 14.1 Calculation of the total field value

Work order

Launch the Microsoft Access DBMS programme and open the database you created in the previous lesson.

1. In the Students table, use a query to calculate the total value for the *Scholarship* and *Overhead* fields.

2. To calculate the field totals, create a query in the *Builder* and select the *Stipend and Overhead* fields in the query form.

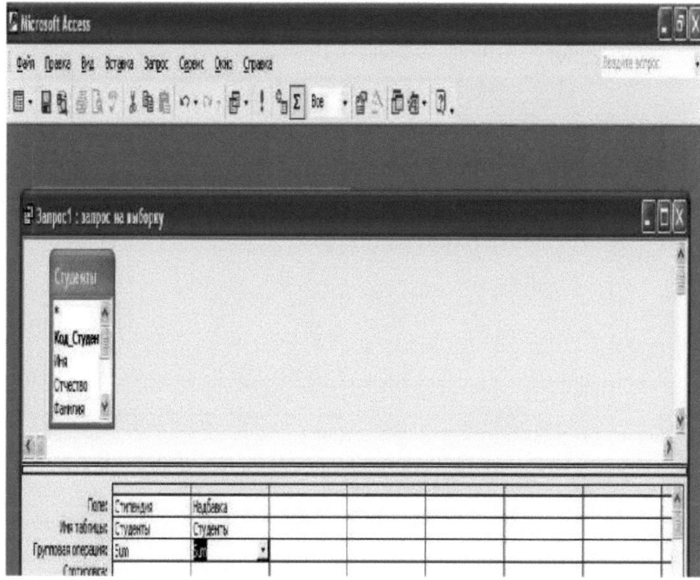

Fig. 14.1. Calculation of the total value for the fields *Scholarship* and *Overhead*

3. Click the *Group Operations* button (Σ) on the toolbar. In the "Group operations" line of the request form that appears, select the Sum function from the drop-down list (Fig. 14.1). Run the query run. Save

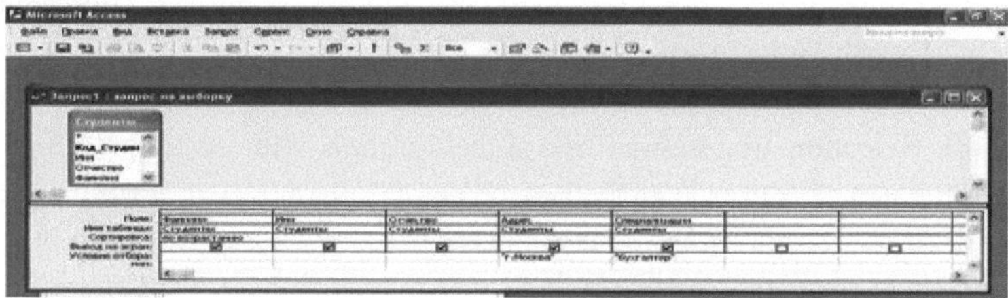

query named "Query - Amount".

Task 14.2. Query for selection in a date range

Work order

1. Create a query on the "Students and Assignments" table to select all the students to whom you want to submit term papers (end date) from 01.05.07 to 25.05.07 (Fig. 14.2). Set sorting by *Start date* in ascending order. Save the query under the name "Query -Total".

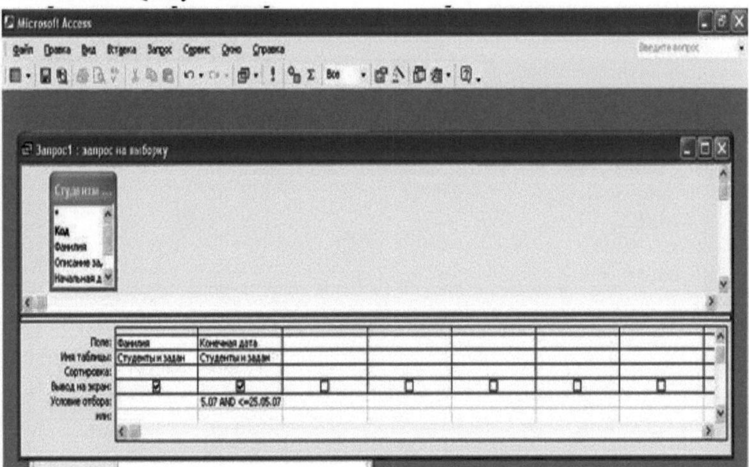

Fig. 14.2. Request for a selection of students who are to submit coursework on the deadline date

Brief Synopsis. The AND logical operator is used to set a condition.

The condition of this query is >= 01.05.07 AND < = 25.05.07.

Task 14.3. Query for selection by several fields Procedure 1. Output in the query all students sorted by surname, studying in the speciality "accountant" and living in Moscow (Fig. 14.3).

Save the request under the name "Accountant-Moscow".

Fig. 14.3. Selection by *Address* and *Specialisation* with sorting by *Surname*

Quick reference. *A report* is a database object designed to output (to the screen, printer or file) information from the database.

Task 14.4 Creating an auto report

Work order

1. Create an auto report to a column on the Students table.

Quick Reference. After selecting a record source and layout (per column, ribbon), AutoReport creates a report that uses all fields of the record source and applies the last used AutoFormat.

2. Select the base object - *Reports.* Click the *Create* button, in the *New Report* window that opens, select the type of report - "Auto Report: per column" (Fig.

14.4).

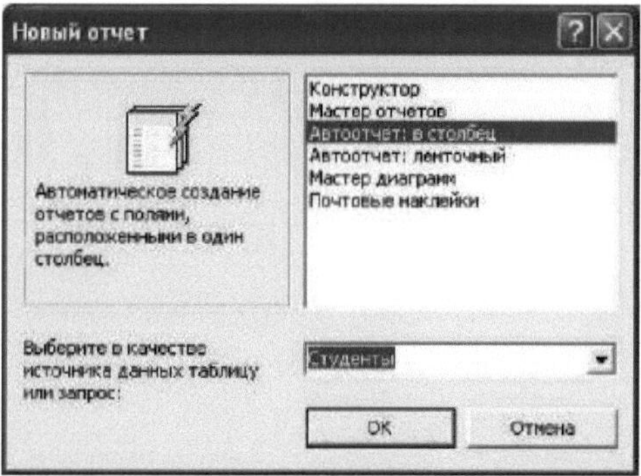

Fig. 14.4. Creating an autoreport to a column

Quick Reference. When selecting the type of auto report, remember that in the ribbon report the field names are arranged in a row like in a table. Several records are placed on each page, which is convenient for viewing and comparing data. However, not all fields can fit in one line, so the ribbon report is inconvenient to use when there are a large number of fields.

3. Select the "Students" table as the data source. Click *OK* and wait for the AutoReport Wizard to finish.

View the report in *Preview* mode *(File/Preview).*

4. Switch to the *Constructor* mode and see how the report looks like in this mode.

5. Save the report under the name "Students".

Task 14.5: Create a report on the "Students and Assignments" table using the Report Wizard

Work order

Quick Reference. The wizard asks detailed questions about record sources, fields, layout, required formats and creates a report based on the answers received.

1. Select the base object - *Reports.* Click the *Create* button, select the Report Wizard report type in the *New* Report window that opens. Select the "Students and assignments" table as the data source, select all fields, set sorting by the field Assignment *description,* layout type - to column.

An example view of the report is shown in Fig. 14.5. Save the report under the name "Students and Assignments".

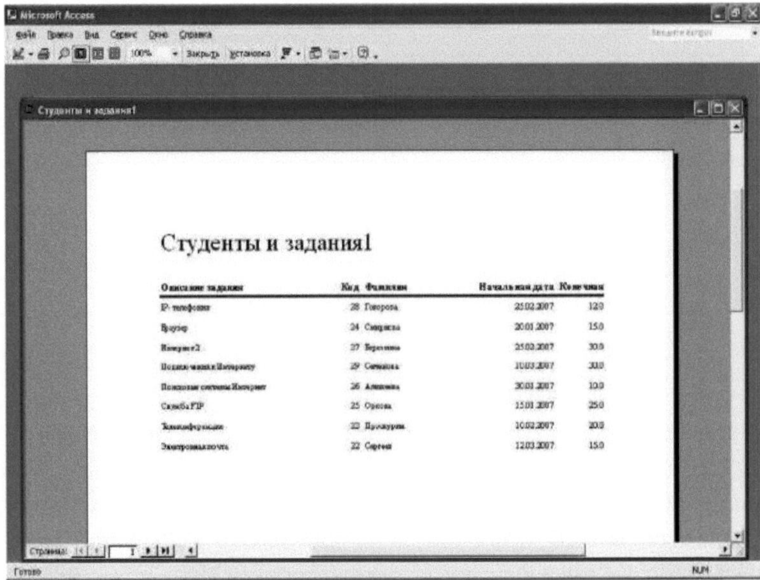

Fig. 14.5. View of the report in a column

Additional tasks

Task 14.6: In the same database in the table "Students" create a new field "Student works" with the logical field type

Work order

1. Create a query to sample students who are working. When creating the query, enter "Yes" in the selection bar of the *Student Working* field.

Brief reference. To create a field with a logical type, open the "Students" table in the *Constructor* mode (Figure 14.6). After that enter the field name and set the logical type of the field.

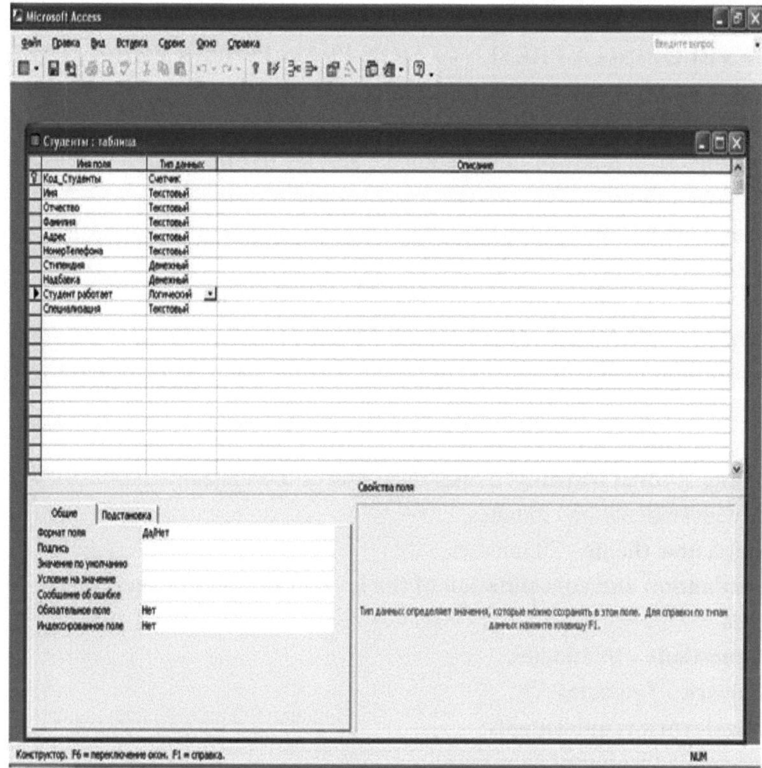

Figure 14. 6. Setting the logical type of the field

2. Go to the normal table view and fill the created table field with data, marking with the mouse about half of the students as working (you will see a tick in the field).

Task 14.7: Using the data from the table "Students", create a query to select non-working students studying in the specialisation "technologist"

Reporting form: When carrying out the practical work, it is necessary to: ý Write down the number and topic of the lesson. ý Write down the task. ý Describe in detail the performance of the work. ý Answer the control questions.

Control Questions:

1. Give the definition of a report.
2. Describe the algorithm for creating a sample query using the wizard.
3. Describe the algorithm for creating a selection query in the constructor mode.
4. What types of reports do you know?
5. Describe the algorithm for creating an auto-report.

Recommended reading: 1.1,1.2, 2.2.

Practical work No. 15

DEVELOPING A PRESENTATION IN MS POWER POINT. TASK EFFECTS AND DEMONSTRATION OF PRESENTATIONS IN MS POWER POINT

Class Objective. Study of information technology of presentation development in MS Power Point.

Type of work: frontal

Lead time: 2 hours

Equipment: PC, Microsoft Power Point

The chronological map of the lesson is 80 minutes.

Organisational part: cleanliness of premises, equipment, sanitary and hygienic conditions.

Student attendance is 2 minutes.

Assessing student learning: a brief overview of the subject,

Q&A with students - 10 minutes.

Setting a new theme - 20 minutes.

Determination and consolidation of the level of mastery of the subject - 35 minutes.

Test questions - 10 minutes.

Homework - 3 minutes.

Practical work requirements:

1. answer the theoretical questions
2. organise the tasks in the practical workbook

Theoretical material

Presentation (from the English word -Presentation!) is a set of coloured pictures - slides on a certain topic. For demonstration, 35-millimetre slides and transparent films are used to show the image on the screen with the help of a projector. Recently, colour LCD panels directly connected to the computer screen have become widespread.

A PowerPoint presentation is a set of slides and special effects that are shown on the screen, handouts, as well as an outline and outline of the report, stored in a single file with the extension RRT. With the help of this programme we can prepare a presentation without using slides, which can then be printed on transparencies, paper, 35-millimetre slides or simply displayed on a computer screen, we can also create an outline of the report and handout material for distribution to the audience.

Quick Reference. You can create a presentation in two ways - manually (without using presets) and using the AutoContent Wizard.

The process of preparing a presentation is divided into three stages: direct development of the presentation (design of each slide); preparation of handouts and demonstration of the presentation.

Steps in creating a presentation

1. The topic of the future presentation is Microsoft Office programmes learnt.
2. The number of slides is 5 slides.
3. Slide structure: 1st slide - cover page;

2, Slides 3, 4, 5 are devoted to MS Word, MS Excel, MS Access, MS Power Point programmes.

Task 15.1 Create a presentation title slide

Work order

1. Start the Microsoft Power Point programme. To do this, in a standard MS Office installation, run *Start/Programs/Microsoft Power Point.* In the opened Power Point window, designed to open or select a presentation, in the group of fields select *Create a presentation using* select *Empty presentation* and click *OK* (Fig. 15.1).

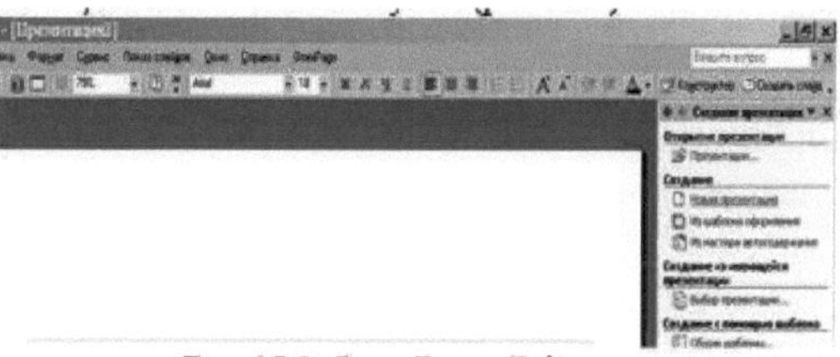

Fig. 15.2. Creating a slide using the layout

2. *3.* Select the very first type - title slide (the first sample on the left in the top row). The first slide will appear on the screen with markup for text entry (filler marks) (Fig. 15.3). Set the screen to normal view *(View/Ordinary).*

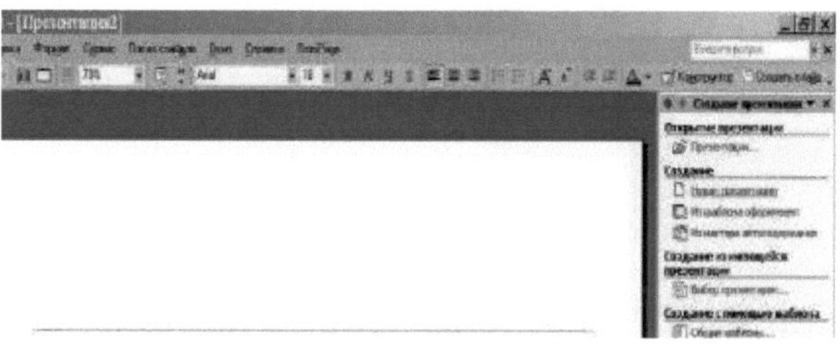

Fig. 15.1. Power Point window

3. The next step is to display the *Create Slide* window, *which* shows various options for slide layout (Fig.15.2).

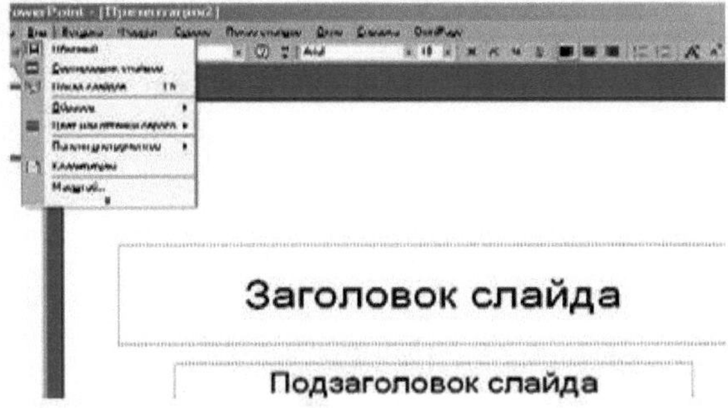

Fig.15.3. Slide with markup for text input

Quick Reference. Filler marks are frames with a dotted outline that appear when you create a new slide. These frames serve as placeholders for text, tables, charts, and graphs. To add text to a placeholder marker, you click and enter text, and to enter an object, you double-click.

4. Explore the programme interface by moving the mouse to different elements of the screen.

5. Select the colour design of the slides using the design design templates *(Format/Slide Layout/Design Templates)* (Fig. 15.4).

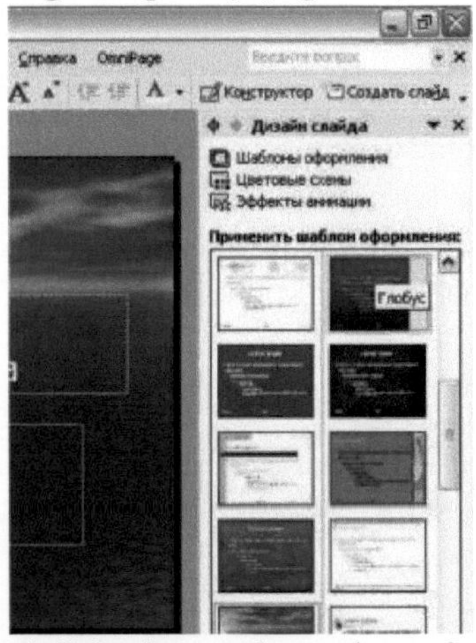

Fig. 15.4. Selecting a colour scheme for slides

6. Enter from the keyboard the text of the heading - Microsoft Office and the sub-heading - Summary of the programmes studied.

To do this, just click on the filler label and enter the text, which will be automatically formatted in accordance with the settings of the selected template (Fig. 15.5).

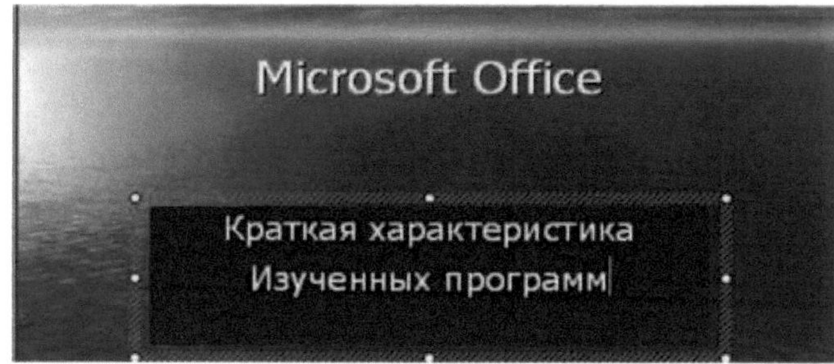

Fig. 15.5. Presentation cover page

7. Save the created file with the name "My Presentation" in your folder with the command *File/Save.*

Task 15.2 Create the second slide of the presentation - text with a list Work order

1. Execute *the Insert/New Slide* command. Select Auto Layout - second left sample in the top row (labelled list) and click *OK.*
2. In the top line, enter the name of the programme "MS Word text editor".
3. In the lower frame, enter the text as a list. Clicking on a placeholder label allows you to enter a bulleted list. Move to a new paragraph by pressing the [Enter] key.

Sample text

The text editor allows you to:

- create text documents;
- formatting text and paragraphing in documents;
- enter footers in a document;
- create and format tables;
- design lists in text documents;
- present text in multiple columns;
- insert pictures into the document;
- prepare the document for printing.

4. Perform the current file save.

Task 15.3 Create a third slide of the presentation - two-column text

Work order

1. Execute the Insert/New Slide command . Select Auto markup - text in two columns and click OK.
2. In the upper line enter the name of the programme "MS Excel Tabular Processor". If necessary, reduce the font size.
3. Enter the content in the columns. Clicking on a column's placeholder label allows you to enter text into the column.

Sample text

Tabular processor capabilities:

1 column:

- entering data into cells;
- autocomplete cells;
- settlement organisation;
- plotting and formatting diagrams;
- use of functions in calculations;

2 column

- application of relative and absolute addressing;
- data sorting;
- data filtering and conditional formatting.

4. Perform the current file save.

Task 15.4: Create the fourth slide of the presentation - text with a table

Work order

1. Execute *the Insert/New Slide* command. Select Auto Layout - the first right sample in the top row (text with table) and click *OK.*

2. Enter the programme name "MS Access DBMS" in the upper line. If necessary, change the font size.

3. Double-click in the lower frame - the window of data table parameters setting will appear. Set the number of columns - 2, rows - 5.

4. In the table that appears, merge the cells in the first row of the table and fill them using the toolbar.

5. Enter the initial data presented in Table 1. For convenience, open the "Tables and Boundaries" toolbar *(View/Toolbars).*

Table 1.

Database design	
Tables	data storage
Forms	for data entry
Enquiries	data management
Reports	to enter information from the database

6. Perform the current save f ayla.

Task 15.5: Create the fifth slide of the presentation - text with a picture

Work order

1. Execute *the Insert/New Slide* command. Select Auto Layout - the first sample on the left in the bottom row (text and graphics) and click *OK.*
2. Enter the name of the programme "MS Power Point" in the top line. If necessary, change the font size.

3. In the left frame, type the text in the pattern. Align the text to the right.

MICROSOFT POWER POINT

Sample text

In most cases, the presentation is prepared to be shown using a computer, because it is in this way of showing the presentation that all the advantages of an electronic presentation can be realised.

4. In the right frame, enter a drawing by double-clicking on the right frame intended for inserting a drawing.
5. Re-colour the drawing. To do this, click the drawing to select it (small squares appear on the sides of the drawing) and click the *Change drawing colour* button in the *Image Adjustment* panel. You can select a new colour for each colour used in the drawing. The colour changes will be displayed in the preview window. When you are finished, click *OK*.
6. By clicking on the slide, remove the marker-squares of the drawing, perform the current file saving by pressing [Ctrl]+[S].

Task 15.6 Change the style of headings

To do this, run the *View/Sample/Sample Slides* command. Click on the title, change the font type (use Arial Cyr instead of Times New Roman or vice versa).

Task 15.7: Applying animation effects

Work order

1. Place the cursor on the first slide. Place the cursor on the first slide. To set the animation, highlight the title and execute *the Slide Show/Animation Setup* command. Set the animation customisation options (select the effect - flying to the left). You can use the right-click context menu to call the *Animation* Setup window.
2. Apply an animation effect to the title of the second slide - appearing on top of the words. Apply different animation effects to the titles of the other slides.
3. To view the animation effect, perform a slide show by executing *the View/Slide Show* command or pressing the [F5] key.

Task 15.8: Set the slide transition method.

Work order

1. The slide transition method determines how a new slide will appear in a presentation.
2. From the *Slide Show* menu, select the *Slide Change* command.
3. From the Transition Effects drop-down list, browse through the available options. Select:

effect - vertical blinds (medium);

the sound is bells;

advancement - automatically after 5 s.

Once you have selected all the slide change options, click on the *Apply to All* button.

4. To view the slide transition method, perform a slide demonstration by executing the command *View/Slide Show* or
press the [F5] key.

Task 15.9: Include the date/time and slide number in the slide

Work order

1. To include a slide number in the slide, execute *the Insert/Slide Number* command. Agree to switch to the footer and in the opened *Columns* window (Fig. 28.3) tick the *Slide Number* box.
2. To include the date/time in the slide in the same window
Columns tick *Auto Update* and *Date/Time* with the mouse.
3. Click the *Apply to All* button.
4. Execute the automatic slide show and close the presentation.

Additional tasks

Assignment 15.10 Create a presentation about the students in your study group Quick Reference. It is convenient to copy slides of the same type. If you set the slide transition settings before copying, all new slides will already have the corresponding settings.

Reporting Form:

When carrying out practical work, it is necessary to :
Write down the number and topic of the class.
Write down the assignment.
Describe the performance of the work in detail.
Answer the control questions.

Supervisory Questions:

1. Give a definition of a presentation.
2. What is the MICROSOFT POWER POINT programme designed for?
3. How do I set animations for slides?
4. What is the process for displaying presentations?

Recommended reading: 1.1,1.2,1.4, 2.2.

Literature

1. Mandatory

1. Lyakhovich V.F. Fundamentals of Informatics: textbook / V.F. Lyakhovich, S.O. Kramarov. - Rostov-on-Don: Phoenix, 2010. - 540 c.
2. Mikheeva E.V. Practicum in Informatics: textbook / E.V. Mikheeva. 4th edition, stereotype. - Moscow: Academy, 2011. - 187 c.
3. Mogilev A. V. Mogilev A.V. Mogilev: Textbook for students. A.V. Mogilev, N.I. Pak, E.K. Henner. - Moscow: Academy, 2009.- 880 p.
4. Popov, E.B. Fundamentals of computer technologies: textbook / E.B. Popov. Popov. - Moscow: Finance and Statistics, 2010. - 703 c.

2. More

1. Kolmykova E.A. Informatics: textbook / E.A. Kolmykova, I.A. Kumskova. - Moscow: Academia, 2010. - 414 c.
2. Sergeeva I.I. Informatics: textbook / I.I. Sergeeva, A.A. Muzalevskaya, N.V. Tarasova. - M.: FORUM-INFRA - M, 2011. - 335 c.

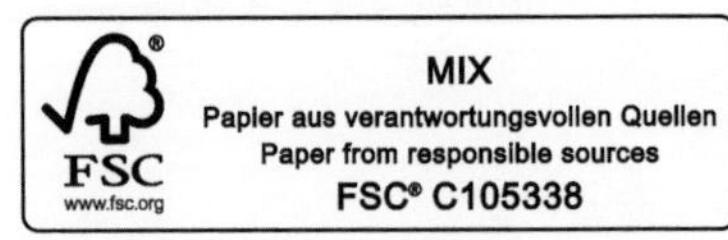

Printed by Books on Demand GmbH, Norderstedt / Germany